Attention and Responsibility in Global Health

Attention and Responsibility in Global Health shows the construction of health through what is neglected and how the label of neglect is used to make the case that a shift in attitudes towards tropical diseases is based on changing policy practices of health and disease.

Tropical diseases have moved from being of high importance for European empires to being neglected and unknown, and then returning to the spotlight once again. During this process, the understanding, framing, and overall character of the disease grouping has changed through a rediscovery of a health issue once rendered neglectable. The book depicts this change in relevance of tropical diseases from colonial history to the present day diseases across political, cultural, and socio-economic contexts. It shows the transformation of tropical diseases as a grouping that uncovers the changing strategies, tactics, and unintended consequences of advocacy campaigning by scientists, NGOs, and policymakers to drive disease issues up the policy agenda.

Drawing on the emergent field of ignorance studies, the book explores ideas about the uses and deployment of both strategic and unintentional "not knowing". It is aimed at academics and students in science and technology studies, the sociology of health and medicine, environmental sociology, public policy, and the history of science.

Samantha Vanderslott is a University Research Lecturer at Oxford Vaccine Group, at the University of Oxford. She studies health and society topics with a focus on neglected tropical diseases, outbreak responses, and public attitudes to vaccines.

Routledge Research in Ignorance Studies

This timely series brings together cutting-edge scholarship in the emergent field of studies on the flipside of knowledge. It addresses the blossoming interest – within an increasing number of disciplines – in the uses and deployment of strategic not knowing, the right to non-knowledge, of forgetting, of producing, and keeping secrets.

From classical perspectives on the unknown to the most recent analyses in theology, brain research, decision-making, economics, political science, and science and technology studies, this interdisciplinary series will serve as an indispensable resource for both students and scholars. The *Routledge Research in Ignorance Studies* series places the study of ignorance in historical and interdisciplinary context.

Series editors:

Matthias Gross is Professor and Head of the Department of Urban and Environmental Sociology, Helmholtz Centre for Environmental Research, UFZ, Leipzig, Germany.

Linsey McGoey is Senior Lecturer in Sociology at the University of Essex.

Michael Smithson is a Professor in the Research School of Psychology at The Australian National University.

Ignorance and Change
Anticipatory Knowledge and the European Refugee Crisis
Adriana Mica, Anna Horolets, Mikołaj Pawlak, and Paweł Kubicki

Attention and Responsibility in Global Health
The Currency of Neglect
Samantha Vanderslott

For more information about the series, please visit: www.routledge.com/Routledge-Research-in-Ignorance-Studies/book-series/RRIGS

Attention and Responsibility in Global Health

The Currency of Neglect

Samantha Vanderslott

Routledge
Taylor & Francis Group

LONDON AND NEW YORK

First published 2022
by Routledge
2 Park Square, Milton Park, Abingdon, Oxon OX14 4RN

and by Routledge
605 Third Avenue, New York, NY 10158

Routledge is an imprint of the Taylor & Francis Group, an informa business

© 2022 Samantha Vanderslott

The right of Samantha Vanderslott to be identified as author of this work has been asserted by her in accordance with sections 77 and 78 of the Copyright, Designs and Patents Act 1988.

British Library Cataloguing-in-Publication Data
A catalogue record for this book is available from the British Library

Library of Congress Cataloging-in-Publication Data
Names: Vanderslott, Samantha, author.
Title: Attention and responsibility in global health: the
currency of neglect / Samantha Vanderslott.
Description: Milton Park, Abingdon, Oxon; New York, NY: Routledge, 2021. |
Series: Routledge research in ignorance studies |
Includes bibliographical references and index.
Identifiers: LCCN 2021009426 (print) | LCCN 2021009427 (ebook) |
ISBN 9780367376536 (hardback) | ISBN 9781032060767 (paperback) |
ISBN 9780429355448 (ebook)
Subjects: LCSH: Public health. | Health attitudes. |
Research. | World health–Case studies.
Classification: LCC RA441 .V36 2021 (print) |
LCC RA441 (ebook) | DDC 362.1–dc23
LC record available at https://lccn.loc.gov/2021009426
LC ebook record available at https://lccn.loc.gov/2021009427

ISBN: 978-0-367-37653-6 (hbk)
ISBN: 978-1-032-06076-7 (pbk)
ISBN: 978-0-429-35544-8 (ebk)

Typeset in Times New Roman
by Newgen Publishing UK

For my family, Vanderslotts and Pradelskis.

Contents

Illustrations

Acknowledgements

My PhD supervisors Brian Balmer and Jack Stilgoe guided me in the ideas behind this book while working on my thesis in Science and Technology Studies at UCL and this final product was improved through the input of my examiners Tiago Mata and Catherine Will. I continue to have thanks for the many interviewees who took the time to speak and include me in the world of neglected tropical diseases, and also Sarah and Michael Marks who helped me arrange interviews. I am grateful for the research stays during my PhD: through the snowy Cambridge winter with Sheila Jasanoff, director of Program on Science, Technology, and Society at Harvard University, the sunny Valencia INGENIO PhD days, and the Brocher Foundation on Lake Geneva. I was inspired through these wonderful places of academic exchange. Over the last few years, I am glad to have found a conducive environment at the University of Oxford and the support and encouragement of Andrew Pollard, director of the Oxford Vaccine Group, as well as through the Collective Responsibility for Infectious Disease programme at the Oxford Martin School. While working on attitudes to vaccination, I have been able to further develop my thoughts about concepts of attention, neglect, and responsibility in global health. My colleagues Claas Kirchhelle, Tonia Thomas, and Nina Hallowell have been especially helpful in discussions on these topics. Enthusiasm from the editors of the Ignorance Studies Series, especially Matthias Gross, and at Routledge Emily Briggs and Lakshita Joshi, meant that this book went from idea to reality. My family, as always, have been supportive throughout. Any errors are of course, my own.

Funding

My PhD was funded by an Economic and Social Research Council Studentship upon which this research was based [grant number ES/J500185/1].

Abbreviations

APOC	African Programme for Onchocerciasis Control
APPMG	The All-Party Parliamentary Group on Malaria and Neglected Tropical Diseases
BMGF	Bill and Melinda Gates Foundation
CDC	Centers for Disease Control and Prevention
CL	Cutaneous leishmaniasis
CTD	WHO Division of Control of Tropical Diseases
DALYs	Disability-adjusted life years
DEC	Diethylcarbamazine
DFID	UK Department for International Development
DNDi	Drugs for Neglected Diseases Initiative
DW	Disability weights
EBA	Evidence-based advocacy
EBM	Evidence-based medicine
EBPM	Evidence-based policymaking
ECDC	European Centre for Disease Prevention and Control
FDA	Food and Drug Administration
GAVI	Global Alliance for Vaccines and Immunization
GBD	Global Burden of Disease
GFATM	The Global Fund to Fight AIDS, Tuberculosis and Malaria
G-FINDER	Global Funding of Innovation for Neglected Diseases Survey
GHI	Global Health Initiative
GND	Great Neglected Diseases of Mankind
HAT	Human African trypanosomiasis
IR	International relations
LSE	London School of Economics and Political Science
LSHTM	London School of Hygiene and Tropical Medicine
LSTM	Liverpool School of Tropical Medicine
MDA	Mass drug administration
MDG	Millennium Development Goal
MDT	Multi-drug therapy

ML	Mucocutaneous leishmaniasis
MSF	Médecins Sans Frontières
NCDs	Non-communicable diseases
NGO	Non-governmental organisation
NTDs	Neglected tropical diseases
PEPFAR	President's Emergency Plan for AIDS Relief
QALYs	Quality-adjusted life years
R&D	Research and development
RCT	Randomised controlled trial
TB	Tuberculosis
TDR	The Special Programme for Research and Training in Tropical Diseases
'The big 3'	AIDS/HIV, TB, and malaria
SAFE	Surgery, antibiotics, facial cleanliness, and environmental improvement
SCI	The Schistosomiasis Control Initiative
SDG	Sustainable Development Goal
Swiss TPH	Swiss Tropical and Public Health Institute
UN	United Nations
USAID	US Agency for International Development
VL	Visceral leishmaniasis
WASH	Water, sanitation, and hygiene
WB	World Bank
WHO	World Health Organization

Part I

Becoming neglected

Chapter 1

Introduction

Caring about neglected narratives

Uncovering the neglected

Postcolonial and feminist literature has had a long-held concern with 'the other'. As Hephzibah Anderson explains, these subversive points of view have produced: "... intriguing new insights into classic works of fiction ... by giving voice to the marginalised and the maligned" (2016). It is not my intention to 'give voice' to these marginalised and maligned, which is better fulfilled by others, particularly anthropologists.[1] However, as with literary theory, neglected aspects of texts are being revisited, and critics are appraising what this means for literary study. Observing how the phenomenon of neglect is perceived and enacted within policy has a similar value, to reveal aspects of competition and congruity within policymaking. This book specifically explores the nature of neglect in policy through neglected tropical diseases (NTDs), drawing on the growing ignorance studies literature. Such recent scholarship has begun to care about which policy problems are not currently being addressed but should be, due to being unaware, ignorant, having poor information, or other uncertainties (Frickel, 2014; Harman, 2012; Rappert & Balmer, 2016; Gross & McGoey, 2015). Exploring why some issues and topics are not on policy agendas[2] provides insight into how problems are identified and selected from competing issues.

I have been fortunate to observe the admirable efforts of scientists, NGO workers, and policymakers in trying to make a difference to this state of affairs. I conducted 55 semi-structured interviews with such stakeholders between 2013 and 2016, with a concentration on the USA and UK, as well as two fieldwork trips to Brazil and China. I also undertook a discourse analysis using a wide range of documentary sources. Although it is not the full story about NTDs, I believe the story of these global health actors story is worth telling, and from a critical perspective that goes beyond the biomedical or journalistic accounts that have been written thus far. More than this, I think it is important to understand why problems are characterised through the lens of neglect, and how, as a result, these problems rise in prominence. Names matter – and calling diseases 'neglected' has a meaning and an effect, as Rosenberg eloquently describes: "In some ways disease does not exist until

we have agreed that it does, by perceiving, naming and responding to it ..."
(Rosenberg & Golden, 1992, pp. xiii–xxi).

Specifically, calling something neglected is a way of determining and asserting importance and priority. In a competitive global health environment, where donors want to differentiate themselves, the neglected terminology carries a weight of urgency, and of making a difference. It is a paradox that an assertion of importance has the effect of spreading recognition of diseases that had not been considered important enough before. The 'packaging' of diseases as an object of neglect, through language and associated ideas, is what I am interested in exploring further. Therefore, *Attention and Responsibility in Global Health* does not present what has been typically put forward by a social science view of NTDs in the past (e.g. a practical framework or model to better fund or incentivise research into NTDs), but aims for a deeper understanding about the policy world in which they originate.

What are neglected tropical diseases?

'Neglected tropical diseases' (NTDs, for short) is a name for a collection of diseases, coined in the early 2000s, that have received growing attention within global health. As Koplan et al. describe, "(G)lobal health is derived from public health and international health, which, in turn, evolved from hygiene and tropical medicine" (2009, p. 1993). NTDs have gone full circle, originally being largely diseases of hygiene and tropical medicine, to be sidelined on many levels (scientifically, financially, socially, and politically), and now they are of central interest within global health. These 20 diseases are listed by the World Health Organization (WHO) as shown in Box 1.1, in alphabetical order (WHO, 2016a).

The WHO groups NTDs on the basis of agreed common characteristics – just as was done for tropical diseases in former times, but the methods behind the standardising of this grouping are far from straightforward. The various lists of NTDs attest to this difficulty, and I will go into more detail about lists and the politics of categorisation in Chapter 2. For now, it is worth remarking that the 20 NTDs listed by the WHO tend to be the most well acknowledged, and other organisations draw a shorter selection from this list. This is especially the case for organisations running programmes that require direct interventions.[3]

Returning to the WHO's list of 20, the diseases included form a mixed bag of not very pronounceable names, some of which may be familiar to western audiences. Leprosy and rabies are ancient diseases of the poor (Little, 2007). While travellers can vaccinate against rabies, they may also come across chikungunya, for which there is no vaccine. Still, others may pick up one of the other non-descript 'tropical diseases' from a hot country, although some tropical diseases never were especially tropical, discussed in Chapter 2. Rather than being rare and exotic, NTDs are in fact a common affliction – not only a threat to travellers. They are often debilitating and sometimes deadly for the majority of the world's poorest people. The scale of NTDs for the global

---

Box 1.1 WHO list of NTDs

- Buruli ulcer
- Chagas disease
- Dengue and chikungunya
- Dracunculiasis (guinea-worm disease)
- Echinococcosis
- Foodborne trematodiases
- Human African trypanosomiasis (sleeping sickness)
- Leishmaniasis
- Leprosy (Hansen's disease)
- Lymphatic filariasis
- Mycetoma, chromoblastomycosis and other deep mycoses
- Onchocerciasis (river blindness)
- Rabies
- Scabies and other ectoparasites
- Schistosomiasis
- Snakebite envenoming
- Soil-transmitted helminthiases
- Taeniasis/cysticercosis
- Trachoma
- Yaws (endemic treponematosis)

---

poor is large, with one or more NTDs affecting over a billion people in 149 countries (World Health Organization. Department of Control of Neglected Tropical Diseases 2017). Therefore, despite the label of neglect, and perhaps unfamiliarity in the western world, these diseases are widespread and pervasive.

Progress is being made to tackle NTDs, with 'Big Pharma' mostly behind the over $5 billion in drugs donated (ibid.) and global health commitments made through 'The London Declaration' in 2012 and Sustainable Development Goals (SDGs) in 2015, with national NTD master plans coordinated by the WHO. As of 2019, 67 countries implemented preventive chemotherapy (PC), the large-scale delivery of medicines at regular intervals to entire population groups (WHO, 2020), for one out of five diseases, with over one billion individuals receiving treatment for at least one disease, and there have been some strong achievements in elimination (ibid.). For example, Ecuador eliminated onchocerciasis in 2014 (WHO, 2015b), and Vietnam eliminated lymphatic filariasis in 2018 (Dung et al., 2020). These are significant successes in the space of approximately 20 years, seeing as the term 'NTDs' was only coined in the early 2000s. While much more is still to be done, it is remarkable progress.

Considering these diseases have been labelled neglected, especially in terms of global public health awareness and commitments. What then were the events and milestones that led to such an outcome?

Charting a policy history

To explain how progress has been made with NTDs on policy agendas means first pursuing a more fundamental question as to how the new disease grouping arose. NTDs, as a group, reflect how the relative neglect or non-neglect of one issue over another is negotiated through the use of advocacy and measurement. NTDs stand apart from other diseases deemed not neglected – the so-called Big Three, given the name by their advocates as "… three of the deadliest infectious diseases the world has ever known" (Elliott, 2013).

In 2000, HIV/AIDS, tuberculosis (TB), and malaria were causing more than 4 million deaths per year, and the UN's Millennium Development Goals set HIV/AIDS and malaria as a priority (ibid.). In 2002, the Global Fund was set up to tackle these diseases, along with TB, channelling US$4 billion a year in funding. (Global Fund, n.d.). Since then, the Big Three has received the lion's share of attention in policy, media, and academic spheres for being high mortality diseases on a global scale. However, malaria was once a tropical disease, as Kelly and Beisel (2011) note the term 'all except malaria' is shorthand for NTDs. How did malaria become a tropical disease that is *not* neglected?

Kelly and Beisel argue that political concerns and technical capacities have "… transformed malaria into a *global* enemy" (2011, p. 71, emphasis added), despite it being a disease "exclusive to the tropics" (Hamoudi & Sachs, 1999, p. 1). Therefore, malaria, in being a killer disease that has eluded eradication campaigns, becomes a global enemy through a particular 'vision' of a disease as a common concern, requiring global mapping and capital.[4] HIV/AIDS joins malaria, as a newly emergent disease but another global killer, with high death tolls in the high, low-, and middle-income countries; and similarly, TB has historically been a largely global disease affecting all regions (Daniel, 2006).[5]

Competition between diseases is a feature of global health, especially on the grounds of whether the entry to a 'global' category is met or whether a disease is confined to the 'local', from the Big Three competing for attention, followed by NTDs. However, signs of connections across health issues are evident at the WHO: the NTD group has grown, expanding from an original grouping of 13 to 17 to 20; TB joined the HIV/AIDS and malaria group to form the Big Three; and now TB, HIV/AIDS, malaria, NTDs, and hepatitis form a larger cluster. The WHO created this new cluster (that individual disease departments sit under for reporting) in 2015, with the acronym 'HTM' for HIV, tuberculosis, malaria, hepatitis, and NTDs (WHO, 2016a). Since NTDs have risen up policy agendas, they are increasingly referred to along with HIV/AIDs, TB, and malaria as 'the gang of four' in the global health community (Elliott, 2013).

The question remains as to how NTDs reached a similar status as the Big Three. Through the course of this book, by charting the policy development for NTDs, I argue that the use of the term 'neglect' matters in how NTDs gained attention. Assumptions about the conceptual origin of NTDs as a disease grouping initially point to the WHO. The WHO positions itself as the strategic authority on global health policy, to standardise disease groupings through their authority and expertise (Ng & Ruger, 2011). However, a socio-historical analysis reveals an alternative institutional heritage and organisational agency. This analysis aims to understand the role and positioning of global health actors in the struggle for prominence amongst health issues. Pinpointing how neglect has been used involves exploring the conceptual history of NTDs in how neglect has been deployed as a policy rationale, through forms of advocacy and measurement.

Advocacy and measurement tend to be treated separately within global health and public policy more widely. Indeed, a number of studies attest to this separation (see Majone, 1989; Obermeyer, 2003), while research on social movements leans towards questions of politics and advocacy rather than measurement. Advocacy is the support or recommendation for a particular cause, the mode of which is argumentative, to make a case in order to spur action. Research on measurement often covers the role of metrics and provision of evidence. The type of measurement relied on for NTD advocacy is shown through metrics, and also what metrics are able to do beyond direct measurement. The type of measurement of interest dominating in global health is described as objective, scientific, and quantitative.

It is not often that advocacy and measurement go hand in hand as a research topic; rather, features of tension or instrumentality are highlighted. For example, Kapilashrami et al. (2015) examine the tensions between public health evidence collected through various measures and advocacy. They ask whether practitioners and researchers who belong to the traditional 'evidence-based public health paradigm' can lead improvements in public health by being more involved in politics and advocacy (Kapilashrami et al., 2015). To produce evidence through measurement has a legitimising authority, leading to an overemphasis in public health, with the reassurance of objectivity and corporeality thought to sit outside of political manoeuvring through advocacy or other means to be viewed in a neutral fashion (Smith, 2013). Neutrality is at the heart of the distinction – that advocacy cannot be neutral as it is arguing for one side over another.

The case is also made for the instrumental use of advocacy and evidence. Tillman et al. (2014) argue for the advocacy of 'evidence-based measures' to improve society's health, observing that there should be a 'bolder analysis of public health issues' by institutions. The pursuit of evidence can also be led by advocacy as seen with the work of AIDS activists. Epstein has demonstrated that AIDS advocacy groups required the mastering of science to form an 'alternative basis of expertise' in which to acquire and use evidence for advocacy (Epstein, 1996). The use of evidence *for* advocacy has been coined as 'evidence-based advocacy' (EBA), a term that rapidly emerged in the early 2000s. As Storeng and Béhague put it: "This term was used to highlight the importance of persuading the broader global health community to invest in maternal health not by making explicit moral claims, but by using quantitative objective evidence" (2014, p. 261).

EBA has been used by maternal health advocates to 'bolster authority' in public health but can also lead to a technocratic narrowing of policy agendas, borrowing from an 'audit- and business-orientated ethos' (ibid.). In the global maternal health campaigning, EBA signalled a shift from advocacy relying on principled arguments – for example, through a human rights approach that emphasised social justice. Evidence is applied instrumentally through 'creative epidemiology', in modifying the presentation of statistical data[6] depending on the stakeholder audience (Storeng & Béhague, 2014, p. 268). While the use of evidence is explained by Storeng and Béhague, they do not discuss where the evidence comes from and why some types of evidence are produced and others not.

Science and Technology Studies (STS) has shown how both concepts of evidence and advocacy are contested. Evidence, as described by Nowotny, intends to bring "… to the fore what is there to be seen. But not everything that can be made to be seen is admitted as evidence" (2007, p. 481). This description of evidence speaks to the availability and presentation of information and knowledge, with a hierarchy of evidence from the more scientific, measurable, and objective at the top, moving to anecdotal, opinion-based, and subjective at the bottom – more akin to advocacy (Moore & Stilgoe, 2009). Lambert calls the legitimacy instilled by statistical evidence the 'new regime of truth' (2009, p. 17). Evidence acts as proof and justification for why we should care, while advocacy is thought to rely more on moral and ideological argument.

How does advocacy and measurement in the production of argument and evidence relate to neglect? Arguments pertain to the lack of advocacy and measurement as being a cause of neglect. If measurement is of poor quality and scope it can lead to what is referred to as an 'evidence trap' in a self-reinforcing circle of neglect through low resource allocation (Storeng & Béhague, 2014). Advocacy can be a moral obligation, with some scholars arguing that the lack of advocacy is a type of neglect in itself (Kapilashrami et al., 2015, p. 1). Others have argued that advocacy for NTDs is legitimised by a moral characterisation of neglect:

> A pragmatic consequence of this moral sense of 'neglect' is that it legitimises the prominent use of advocacy as a key strategy to address

NTDs, thus legitimising non-governmental organisations' (NGOs) and other actors' (from civil society to philanthropic entities) participation in the political field.

(Jackson & Stephenson, 2014, p. 998)

I intend to go beyond the view that advocacy is a source of tension in using measurement and that measurement in the production of evidence is used 'for' advocacy, as described by Storeng and Béhague (2014); or, in other words, the view that advocacy is needed to 'present evidence'. I will argue that measurement can be a form of advocacy in itself, drawing upon the literature on social movements, social policy, evidence-based policy, and health metrics. Therefore, measuring and provision of metrics acts as advocacy for a cause.

Has NTD research been neglected?

A wider question of neglect pertains to not only neglect in advocacy and measurement but for NTDs as a research focus, in: (1) the lack of social science research on NTDs; (2) the approach that has dominated in researching NTDs (and why this has been the case); (3) which approaches could be beneficial to the study of NTDs; (4) situating the study of these diseases in a policy context by addressing the meaning of 'policy'. I also briefly discuss the adoption of the NTD term in medical and healthcare literature.

Firstly, social science (and in particular, policy) research on NTDs has been lacking. There have been review articles (Allotey et al., 2010; Manderson et al., 2009), an introductory thematic series (of four papers) on NTDs (Allotey, Reidpath, & Pokhrel, 2010) and a series applying a biosocial approach to NTDs focusing on individual NTDs (Parker, Polman, & Allen, 2016). A number of actors from scientists (Hotez, 2013) to NGOs (Agler & Crigler, 2019) have published their accounts of advocacy. Even though the amount and range of NTD research are rising, NTD research from a social science and policy perspective has been restricted to a limited number of studies (Barry, 2014; De Maio, Llovet, & Dinardi, 2014; Mantilla, 2011; Aya Pastrana et al. 2020). Mantilla even charges a collusion of social science in the "low priority and invisibility of NTDs" (2011, p. 118).

While there has been an enormous amount of research on tropical diseases and fledging research on NTDs, these two literatures should now be viewed together. For example, John Farley in his historical works on bilharzia or schistosomiasis (2003) and the International Health Division of the Rockefeller Foundation (2004) explores the connection between health, the economy, and philanthropy, bringing in socio-political accounts, which has wider implications for the study of NTDs. NTDs form a research topic identified to potentially benefit from 'social science' and 'interdisciplinary research' in reaction to a predominately biomedical lens. As described by Reidpath, Allotey, and Subhash:

> These diseases represent a rich and dynamic interplay between vector, host and pathogen which occurs within social, physical and biological contexts. The overwhelming sense, however, is that neglected tropical diseases research is a biomedical endeavour largely excluding the social sciences.
>
> (2011, p. 1)

Particularly the 'intense' advocacy that has brought attention to NTDs is noted as a point to explore further: "... a systematic analysis of this process would make an important contribution to our understanding of advocacy and the dynamic research-policy-practice nexus in public health" (Manderson et al., 2009). Therefore, advocacy has been presented as a key aspect for why NTDs have gained policy attention; but, through the course of this research, I also found that measurement played a similarly important role – advocacy and measurement both fall under a policy understanding of NTDs.

Secondly, the types of theoretical gaps caused by a lack of social science, especially investigator-driven[7] and interdisciplinary research on NTDs, have been highlighted by Reidpath et al. (2011), using bibliometric analysis. They argue that the social science research that has tended to accompany NTD research is either a misclassification of pure clinical research or 'handmaiden' research to support the implementation of biomedical solutions (2011, p. 1). What this dominance has resulted in is a lack of interdisciplinary focus on the "... complex social, cultural, biological and environmental dynamic involved in human pathogenesis" (ibid.). Reidpath et al. locate a systemic bias to this situation in funding that requires "... more sophisticated funders and priority setters who are not beguiled by uncritical biomedical promises ... *designed to support (and never challenge) the curative activities of biomedical research*" (pp. 1–8, emphasis added). De Maio, Llovet, and Dinardi are not very optimistic to see any change, because of a funding bias that "... may continue to prohibit the social sciences from playing anything but a marginal role in interdisciplinary teams" (2014, p. 373).

Thirdly, De Maio (2014), in reiterating that more needs to be done from the perspective of social science, points towards the scarcity of sociological or anthropological accounts of NTDs beyond two classic works concentrating on one NTD – Chagas disease, by Roberto Briceño-León and Gabaldón (1990) and Joseph Bastien (1998). De Maio particularly encourages engagement by sociologists, contending that they have not been involved with the scholarly discussion surrounding NTDs, such that: "... the framing of NTDs has been overly narrow, and a situation that is perhaps best understood as a manifestation of structural violence has instead been seen through a technical rather than socio-political lens" (ibid.).

The social science critiques of the current NTD literature thus far have tended to focus on a dichotomy between the socio-political structural aspect of NTDs and technical medical interventions. It is a dichotomy perhaps overemphasised because a broadly constructivist theoretical approach can still recognise that the problem of NTDs arises from an ideational *and* material basis (Ruggie, 1998). Such an approach that could be described more specifically as co-productionist, in which natural and social orders produce one another (Jasanoff, 2004). The notable exception in considering ideational and material factors is De Maio, who sees the progress for NTDs (in advocacy and success of resources being redirected) as falling across three areas: "... epidemiological indicators, research activity and policy attention" (2014, p. 97). This book follows similar themes but takes a more encompassing outlook through a concentration on advocacy, measurement, and the concept of neglect in policy by ascertaining what advocacy and measurement mean, as modes of positioning NTDs as a new disease grouping characterised by neglect. Both aspects of the technical and socio-political are important in understanding neglect to make the connection with colonial tropical diseases and the policy development of NTDs.

Finally, it is worth noting, early on, that the use of 'policy' in this book describes a directed activity of a diverse group of actors towards a perceived problem. Policy is directed by actors extending further than government, but it still means a rationale is driving the activity, revealed through dominant discourses and narratives. Such a discussion is part of a theoretical and practical shift from government to governance, where a wider range of actors participate in what was once a more exclusive process of government (Hill & Hupe, 2014, p. 1). This is a broader conception of policy used by Colebatch, in policy being an activity that is "... deliberate and purposeful rather than erratic or random" (1998, pp. 6–72). Policy is more than a set of objectives or guiding principles but standardises and articulates practice in how action is framed, rather than simply described. It is in this sense 'policy' is used throughout to mean the *activity directed to the problem of NTDs* and the activity of most concern being with acknowledgement, attention, and most importantly care, as the opposites of neglect in policy.[8]

This book is split into two parts. The first, 'Becoming neglected', describes the lead up to tropical diseases becoming labelled as neglected. This chapter explores theoretical underpinnings of policy problems from the perspective of a number of disciplines to ask questions about how a policy problem is formed, raised in profile, and the types of solutions that are offered. NTDs present a policy problem that involves a tropical disease history, followed by a reconceptualisation and branding, or a 'repackaging', of the neglected aspect of NTDs. I discuss how problematisation has been understood for policy, drawing attention to innovation being directed towards policy solutions and the disciplinary lens taken to policy problems. By the end of the chapter,

I consider how policy problems are related to global health and how the concept of neglect is positioned within this landscape as a form of non-knowledge.

Identifying non-knowledge is powerful grounds for policy rationales and making a case for advocacy and it is surprising how little importance is applied when, discursively, it is a common starting point for any research, policy, and advocacy cause. The framing of absence used includes 'gaps in the literature' where knowledge has not yet been generated and so requires academic focus; 'market failure' where a lack of market provision justifies government intervention; and various descriptors of problems for advocacy from 'underserved', 'unacknowledged', 'ignored' to 'neglected'; while the role of ignorance has been explored for the production of scientific facts (Smithson, 1989).

Chapter 2 covers the most important milestones for the construction of NTDs and in how the present system of global health governance is disaggregated, from the WHO once dominating policy to a situation of numerous important stakeholders (Patrick, 2014). The chapter concentrates on two early initiatives for NTDs by the Rockefeller Foundation and the WHO as illustrative of the general trends in global health governance and the later conceptualisation of NTDs. I consider the common characteristics for what constitutes an NTD and the criteria or methods of standardising the grouping.

While there is instability in the category boundaries, the reasons and consequences for why some diseases are categorised as being part of one group and others a part of another is important. It matters for attention of the global community, the policy approaches employed, and funding and resources applied. A utilitarian approach to classification, in which systematic classification serves practical needs, has played a large and ongoing role in how to classify the natural world (Stepan, 2001, p. 17). However, classification is a "… social and uncertain process" (Freeman and Frisina, 2010). In medicine, diseases are also classified in terms of the people they afflict, rather than only seeking distinctions based on the intrinsic nature of the disease (Bowker & Star, 1999). It is this element of subjective interpretation that I expand upon in the characterisation of one group of people given by another.

The second part of this book 'Becoming un-neglected' looks at how scientist advocates have provided the advocacy and measurement needed to present NTDs as a case worth caring about. Chapter 3 charts the branding of NTDs by UK and US scientists who became advocates, and how this formed part of an elite advocacy movement. It is also important that this book includes the 'endemic' countries where NTDs are prevalent with the "… constant presence and/or usual prevalence of a disease or infectious agent in a population within a geographic area" (CDC, n.d.). Brazil and China, in particular, are countries with potential to contribute scientifically and strategically to the NTD problem and represent a move away from western dominance.

For Chapter 4, I take stock of how NTD policy development is reflected in public discourse to demonstrate the role that measurement has had in conceptualising the NTD problem. Measurement is a way of caring in global health, and evidence (presented through measurement) has acted as a form of advocacy for raising the profile of NTDs. Chapter 5 revisits the initial questions posed by the introduction and discusses the ways that advocacy and measurement showcase neglect. I argue that neglect is present in policy across typologies of information, thinking, action, and emotion. Such an understanding of neglect in policy has implications for who has responsibility and how the concept is used as a resource in global health. The book concludes by presenting how NTDs might be understood as a fledging area of social science research in both shaping and reflecting major changes in global health policy.

The central aim of this book is to situate the change of NTD disease categorisation, advocacy, measurement, and policy characterisation within more widespread changes in the global health era, just as tropical diseases have been situated within a colonial era. By following the journey of a collection of diseases whose grouping has changed for various reasons, I demonstrate how policy problems grow in salience and respond to a changing institutional and structural environment. *Attention and Responsibility in Global Health* argues that neglect is an important problem characterisation, grounded in knowledge, action, and emotion of why certain diseases are made to matter, and why we care about certain diseases above others.

Notes

1   To a lesser degree, I have given voice to scientists in endemic countries, neglected in media and academic accounts. However, patients whose voices are rarely heard, apart from in soundbites of advocacy campaigns or more comprehensively through anthropological study.
2   I use a standard, succinct definition of policy agendas supplied by Cobb and Elder for the "… range of legitimate concerns meriting the attention of the polity" (Cobb & Elder, 1971, p. 905) but expand the conception from polity and to policy.
3   Organisations with direct NTD interventions are US Agency for International Development (USAID), Centers for Disease Control and Prevention (CDC), the Department for International Development (DFID), The Global Network for Neglected Tropical Diseases, Uniting to Combat NTDs, and Drugs for Neglected Diseases Initiative (DNDi). Only the *PLOS* journal on NTDs has a longer list. Being an academic endeavour, there is more reason to encompass a larger number of diseases to have a wide research scope.
4   The main weapon against malaria from the 1950s onwards was aerial DDT spraying, and as a result, "… epidemiological models came to replace detailed entomological reports, malaria shifted further from a situated illness to a global pandemic" (ibid., p. 76).

5   Due to advancements of treatment and control, TB is now mainly a disease of the global poor, in low- and middle-income countries, with some signs of resurgence in poor communities residing in richer countries (Elliott & Arora, 2011).
6   An example of modifying the presentation of statistical data is presenting to a public audience the number of deaths in pregnancy and childbirth in a low- and middle-income country, compared to high-income countries (ibid.). Global level policy actors may view these deaths as too low compared with other issues, so (as with NTDs) the focus needs to be turned from mortality to morbidity and the combined burden of mothers, children, and newborns.
7   Investigator-driven research is a science policy term where the investigator is the one who designs and implements the study as opposed to being given instructions by someone else (Horizon, 2020, https://ec.europa.eu/programmes/horizon2020/en/h2020-section/excellent-science, accessed 2/4/14).
8   Characteristics of 'attention and care' are the opposite to neglect if defined as the failure to give attention or care (Cambridge Dictionary), and I argue that acknowledgement of the need to care is also required.

References

Agler, E., & M. Crigler. 2019. *Under the Big Tree: Extraordinary Stories from the Movement to End Neglected Tropical Diseases*. https://jhupbooks.press.jhu.edu/title/under-big-tree.
Allotey, P., D. D. Reidpath, & S. Pokhrel. 2010. "Social Sciences Research in Neglected Tropical Diseases 1: The Ongoing Neglect in the Neglected Tropical Diseases." *Health Research Policy and Systems/BioMed Central* 8 (1): 32. https://doi.org/10.1186/1478-4505-8-32.
Anderson, H. 2016. "The Book That Changed Jane Eyre Forever." *BBC Culture*. https://bbc.com/culture/story/20161019-the-book-that-changed-jane-eyre-forever?
Aya Pastrana, N., D. Beran, C. Somerville, O. Heller, J. C. Correia, & L. Suzanne Suggs. 2020. "The Process of Building the Priority of Neglected Tropical Diseases: A Global Policy Analysis." Edited by Deborah Mc Farland. *PLOS Neglected Tropical Diseases* 14 (8): e0008498. https://doi.org/10.1371/journal.pntd.0008498.
Barry, J. A. 2014. "Social Sciences Research on Infectious Diseases of Poverty: Too Little and Too Late?" Edited by Courtney Queen. *PLoS Neglected Tropical Diseases* 8 (6): e2803. https://doi.org/10.1371/journal.pntd.0002803.
Bastien, J. 1998. "The Kiss of Death: Chagas' Disease in the Americas." *Revista Panamericana de Salud Pública* 4 (6). https://doi.org/10.1590/S1020-49891998001200019.
Bowker, G. C., & S. L. Star. 1999. *Sorting Things out: Classification and Its Consequences*. MIT Press.
Briceño-León, R., & A. Gabaldón. 1990. *La Casa Enferma: Sociología de La Enfermedad de Chagas*. Fondo Editorial Acta Científica Venezolana.
Cambridge Dictionary. n.d. "Neglect Meaning in the Cambridge English Dictionary." http://dictionary.cambridge.org/dictionary/english/neglect.
CDC. n.d. "Principles of Epidemiology Lesson 1 – Section 11." https://cdc.gov/ophss/csels/dsepd/ss1978/lesson1/section11.html.
Cobb, R. W., & C. D. Elder. 1971. "The Politics of Agenda-Building: An Alternative Perspective for Modern Democratic Theory." *The Journal of Politics* 33 (4): 892–915. https://doi.org/10.2307/2128415.

Colebatch, H. K. 1998. *Policy*. University of Minnesota Press. https://books.google. com/books?id=dxzLFTfSkAYC&pgis=1.

Daniel, T. M. 2006. "The History of Tuberculosis." *Respiratory Medicine* 100 (11): 1862–70. https://doi.org/10.1016/j.rmed.2006.08.006.

Dung, D. T., V. T. Lam Binh, C. M. Worrell, M. Brady, V. Walsh, A. Yajima, Z. Sifri, & L. M. Fox. 2020. "Evaluation of a Facility-Based Inspection Tool to Assess Lymphedema Management Services in Vietnam." Edited by S. Babu. *PLOS Neglected Tropical Diseases* 14 (10): e0008773. https://doi.org/10.1371/journal. pntd.0008773.

Elliott, R. L. 2013. *Third World Diseases*. Springer.

Elliott, R. L., & K. Arora. 2011. *Third World Diseases*. Springer.

Epstein, S. 1996. *Impure Science: AIDS, Activism, and the Politics of Knowledge*. Vol. 9. University of California Press. https://books.google.com/books?hl=en&lr=&id= kZOso0FMsrMC&pgis=1.

Farley, J. 2003. *Bilharzia: A History of Imperial Tropical Medicine*. Cambridge University Press.

Farley, J. 2004. *To Cast out Disease: A History of the International Health Division of the Rockefeller Foundation (1913–1951)*. Oxford University Press.

Freeman, R., & L. Frisina. 2010. "Health Care Systems and the Problem of Classification." *Journal of Comparative Policy Analysis: Research and Practice* 12 (1–2): 163–78. https://doi.org/10.1080/13876980903076278.

Frickel, S. 2014. "Absences: Methodological Note about Nothing, in Particular." *Social Epistemology* 28 (1): 86–95. https://doi.org/10.1080/02691728.2013.862881.

Global Fund. n.d. "Global Fund Overview – The Global Fund to Fight AIDS, Tuberculosis and Malaria." Accessed March 22, 2016. https://theglobalfund.org/ en/overview/.

Hamoudi, A., & J. Sachs. 1999. *The Changing Global Distribution of Malaria: A Review*. https://pdfs.semanticscholar.org/9292/b8a7855485862cae64f040c86c1410 f8a931.pdf.

Harman, S. 2012. *Global Health Governance*. Routledge. https://books.google.com/ books?id=zuvGBQAAQBAJ&pgis=1.

Hill, M. J., & P. L. Hupe. 2014. *Implementing Public Policy: An Introduction to the Study of Operational Governance*. Sage.

Horizon 2020. n.d. "Excellent Science – European Commission." https://ec.europa.eu/ programmes/horizon2020/en/h2020-section/excellent-science.

Hotez, P. J. 2013. *Forgotten People Forgotten Diseases*. Edited by Peter J. Hotez. American Society of Microbiology. https://doi.org/10.1128/9781555818753.

Jackson, Y., & N. Stephenson. 2014. "Neglected Tropical Disease and Emerging Infectious Disease: An Analysis of the History, Promise and Constraints of Two Worldviews." *Global Public Health* 9 (9): 995–1007. https://doi.org/10.1080/ 17441692.2014.941297.

Jasanoff, S. 2004. "States of Knowledge: The Co-Production of Science and Social Order."

Kapilashrami, A., K. E. Smith, S. Fustukian, M. Eltanani, S. Laughlin, T. Robertson, J. Muir, E. Gallova, & E. Scandrett. 2015. "Social Movements and Public Health Advocacy in Action: The UK People's Health Movement." *Journal of Public Health (Oxford, England)*, June, fdv085. https://doi.org/10.1093/pubmed/fdv085.

Kelly, A. H., & Beisel, U. 2011. Neglected Malarias: The Frontlines and Back Alleys of Global Health. *BioSocieties*, 6 (S1), 71–87. http://doi.org/10.1057/biosoc.2010.42.

Koplan, J. P., T. C. Bond, M. H. Merson, K. S. Reddy, Mario Henry Rodriguez, Nelson K. Sewankambo, Judith N. Wasserheit, et al. 2009. "Towards a Common Definition of Global Health." *Lancet (London, England)* 373 (9679): 1993–95. https://doi.org/10.1016/S0140-6736(09)60332-9.

Lambert, H. 2009. "Evidentiary Truths? The Evidence of Anthropology through the Anthropology of Medical Evidence." *Anthropology Today* 25 (1): 16–20. https://doi.org/10.1111/j.1467-8322.2009.00642.x.

Little, L. K. 2007. *Plague and the End of Antiquity: The Pandemic of 541–750.* Cambridge University Press.

Maio, F. D. 2014. *Global Health Inequities: A Sociological Perspective.* Palgrave Macmillan. https://books.google.com/books?id=Ese9CgAAQBAJ& pgis=1.

Maio, F. G. D. I. Llovet, & G. Dinardi. 2014. "Chagas Disease in Non-Endemic Countries: 'Sick Immigrant' Phobia or a Public Health Concern?" *Critical Public Health* 24 (3): 372–80. https://doi.org/10.1080/09581596.2013.836589.

Majone, G. 1989. *Evidence, Argument, and Persuasion in the Policy Process.* Yale University Press.

Manderson, L., J. Aagaard-Hansen, P. Allotey, M. Gyapong, & J. Sommerfeld. 2009. "Social Research on Neglected Diseases of Poverty: Continuing and Emerging Themes." Edited by I. Agyepong. *PLoS Neglected Tropical Diseases* 3 (2): e332. https://doi.org/10.1371/journal.pntd. 0000332.

Mantilla, B. 2011. "Invisible Plagues, Invisible Voices: A Critical Discourse Analysis of Neglected Tropical Diseases." *Soc Med* 6 (3): 118–27. https://doi.org/10.1080/0098559920140401?NEEDACCESS=TRUE.

Moore, A., & J. Stilgoe. 2009. "Experts and Anecdotes: The Role of 'Anecdotal Evidence' in Public Scientific Controversies." *Science, Technology & Human Values* 34 (5): 654–77. https://doi.org/10.1177/0162243908329382.

Ng, N. Y., & J. P. Ruger. 2011. "Global Health Governance at a Crossroads." *Global Health Governance.* http://search.ebscohost.com/login.aspx?direct=true&profile=ehost&scope=site&authtype=crawler&jrnl=19392389&AN=64305235&h=lg908ao62gGaJg2IGECbBbkw9xXdFYjJVTXjg6L04ZGEJcjf%2Bk%2BTngy266Y5ZYSPpL2GOcyKCz3JKGlKuxvk8Q%3D%3D&crl=c.

Nowotny, H. 2007. "How Many Policy Rooms Are There?: Evidence-Based and Other Kinds of Science Policies." *Science, Technology & Human Values* 32 (4): 479–90. https://doi.org/10.1177/0162243907301005.

Obermeyer, C. M. 2003. "The Health Consequences of Female Circumcision: Science, Advocacy, and Standards of Evidence." *Medical Anthropology Quarterly* 17 (3): 394–412. https://doi.org/10.1525/MAQ.2003.17.3.394.

Parker, M., K. Polman, & T. Allen. 2016. "Biosocial Approaches to the Control of Neglected Tropical Diseases." *Journal of Biosocial Science* 48 (S1): Si. https://doi.org/10.1017/S0021932016000389.

Patrick, S. 2014. "The Unruled World." Foreign Affairs. 2014. https://foreignaffairs.com/articles/2013-12-06/unruled-world.

Rappert, B., & B. Balmer. 2016. *Absence in Science, Security and Policy: From Research Agendas to Global Strategy.* Springer. https://books.google.com/books?id=S4-kCgAAQBAJ&pgis=1.

Reidpath, D. D., P. Allotey, & S. Pokhrel. 2011. "Social Sciences Research in Neglected Tropical Diseases 2: A Bibliographic Analysis." *Health Research Policy and Systems/ BioMed Central* 9 (1): 1. https://doi.org/10.1186/1478-4505-9-1.

Rosenberg, C. E., & Golden, J. L. eds., 1992. *Framing Disease: Studies in Cultural History*. Rutgers University Press.

Ruggie, J. G. 1998. "What Makes the World Hang Together? Neo-Utilitarianism and the Social Constructivist Challenge." *International Organization* 52 (4): 855–85. https://doi.org/10.1162/002081898550770.

Smith, K. 2013. *Beyond Evidence-Based Policy in Public Health*. Palgrave Macmillan. https://doi.org/10.1057/9781137026583.

Smithson, M. 1989. A Vocabulary of Ignorance. In *Ignorance and Uncertainty* (pp. 1–13). Springer.

Stepan, N. 2001. *Picturing Tropical Nature*. Reaktion Books. https://books.google.com/books?id=tW7dNwfwkPcC&pgis=1.

Storeng, K. T., & D. P. Béhague. 2014. "Playing the Numbers Game: Evidence-Based Advocacy and the Technocratic Narrowing of the Safe Motherhood Initiative." *Medical Anthropology Quarterly* 28 (2): 260–79. https://doi.org/10.1111/maq.12072.

Tillmann, T., P. Baker, T. Crocker-Buque, S. Rana, B. Bouquet, S. C. Davies, M. Marmot, et al. 2014. "Shortage of Public Health Independence and Advocacy in the UK." *The Lancet* 383 (9913): 213. https://doi.org/10.1016/S0140-6736(14)60064-7.

WHO. 2015a. "First WHO Report on Neglected Tropical Diseases: Working to Overcome the Global Impact of Neglected Tropical Diseases." World Health Organization. https://who.int/neglected_diseases/2010report/en/.

———. 2015b. "Investing to Overcome the Global Impact of Neglected Tropical Diseases: Third WHO Report on Neglected Tropical Diseases." http://apps.who.int/iris/bitstream/10665/152781/1/9789241564861_eng.pdf.

———. 2016a. "Accelerating Progress on HIV, Tuberculosis, Malaria, Hepatitis and Neglected Tropical Diseases." World Health Organization. https://who.int/neglected_diseases/diseases/en/, Accessed 2/4/16.

———. 2016b. "The 17 Neglected Tropical Diseases." World Health Organization. 2016. https://who.int/neglected_diseases/diseases/en/.

———. 2020. "Summary of Global Update on Implementation of Preventive Chemotherapy against Neglected Tropical Diseases in 2019." *The Weekly Epidemiological Record* 469–74. https://pesquisa.bvsalud.org/portal/resource/pt/who-334568.

Chapter 2

Theoretical approaches to attention and neglect

Policy problems

What is a problem for policy? And how are evidence and advocacy used to problematise? Problematisation has a well-established intellectual basis through the work of Michel Foucault and scholarship by public policy theorists on how policy problems are constituted, although my use of policy is in a broad sense to include public, private, and philanthropic actors that contribute to policymaking. I begin by discussing how evidence-based policymaking and social movements constitute a large part of how measurement and advocacy are commonly described in policy, as well as the role of innovation in presenting solutions.

Next, I discuss the disciplinary lens in global health. A body of literature has developed charting a new era of 'global health', which is closely tied to governance. Katherine Kelly calls global health the "... preferred label for attempts to govern the health of the global population" (2015). Sophie Harman (2014) describes how new and older institutions, including non-governmental organisations (NGOs) and private philanthropy, have led to a blurred landscape of global health governance, without leadership on how they will work together. Economists, historians, and others from epidemiologists to health economists and anthropologists have also been influential within global public health policy, often as part of interdisciplinary teams.

Problematisation

Early work on problem types[1] in policy was undertaken by political theorists David Rochefort and Roger Cobb (1993) on the broader topic of 'problem definition'. While used interchangeably, issues and problems have different meanings. An issue is a "... dispute between parties in which they join in the hope of arriving at a decision or solution" (Strydom, 1999, p. 71). A divergence of opinion is already assumed, but competing parties have the ambition to reach a decision or solution, while a problem is a matter or situation regarded as "unwelcome or harmful and needing to be dealt with and overcome" (Oxford Dictionaries). It is a recognition that an undesirable situation exists to be resolved, while a second definition is: "... A thing that is difficult to achieve", so a degree of difficulty is already implicit (ibid.). The ability to identify problems, make lists, and prioritise, is determined by how undesirable the situation is and the difficulty or ease of solving – meaning importance, urgency, and solvability are key tenets of what it means to address a problem.

Directing efforts towards identifying and strategising problems concerning the public, society, or humankind, has not always happened in a coordinated or high-level manner. As a famous early instance of listing problems over a century ago, David Hilbert defined a set of 23 unsolved mathematical problems (Floridi, 2004). Problems were listed as 'Grand Challenges', and such a construction would be repeated by other disciplines and also governments, universities, and NGOs. Indeed, a global outlook for policy problems has produced more concerted efforts towards generating challenge lists. The Bill and Melinda Gates Foundation 'revitalised' the concept in 2003 by identifying 14 Grand Challenges in global health and extending funding to $100m (Bill & Melinda Gates Foundation, n.d.). As Bill Gates describes: "By harnessing the world's capacity for scientific innovation, I believe we can transform health in the developing world and save millions of lives" (quoted by Kelly & Beisel, 2011, p. 79).

Listing problems in a goal-orientated way has been viewed by some to represent a techno-scientific optimism. As Kelly and Beisel caution, it is a "... problematic analogy between global health and algebraic puzzles" (2011, p. 79). Global problem lists are, as Isabelle Stengers describes, a continuation of the modernist epoch from "... fifty years ago, when the grand perspectives on techno-scientific innovation were synonymous with progress" – but such confidence has since been shaken (2015, p. 29).

Also, the types of policy problem centre on broad topics, based on spheres that problems inhabit (health, development, environment, welfare). Fewer sources focus on the characteristics describing the nature of problems, in terms of their level of difficulty to solve. Problems can be described by level of difficulty – wicked (not tame), degree of determinability – anticipatory (not established), or amount of attention and care – neglected (not acknowledged). Table 2.1 shows a description of the major types of policy problem, based on common characterisations of solvability and opposite (or alternative) scenarios.

Here we can see where a 'neglected' characterisation might fit in relation to other characterisations and what those different policy treatments mean. It is the case that characterisations follow hype and trends, as certain characterisations are more popularly used at various times than others. The values encompassed relate predominately to how the problem manifests in time and space (local/global or past-looking/future-looking), who is

Table 2.1 Major types of policy problem and opposite scenarios

Type of problem	Opposite scenario	Values	Reference
Wicked			
Weaker/stronger levels of difficulty with super wicked to insoluble, complex, and complicated	Tame, simple, straightforward	Past and future, technical, local and global, everyone	(Rittel & Webber, 1973) (Cairney, 2012) (Ramalingam, 2014)
Anticipatory			
Grades of determinacy from predictive, forecasted to speculative	Established, current, immediate	Future, technical, global	(Anderson, 2010)
Neglected			
Wider/public portrayal low-profile and unrecognised	Prevalent, acknowledged, well-known, high-profile	Political, local, minority groups	(Rappert & Balmer, 2016) (Harman, 2014)

affected (a particular group or everyone) and who is responsible for solutions (depending on a whether it is a technical or political problem). These three problem types are outcome-orientated ways of looking at problems on the grounds of solvability.

Wicked problems are "… difficult or impossible to solve because of incomplete, contradictory, and changing requirements" (Ramalingam, 2014). What is the remedy for difficult or even impossible solvability? Complexity theory has been one proposal developed as a reaction and response to the non-linearity of problems (Goldstein, 1999). As a broad field, which purports to span the natural and social sciences, it is a research approach that has taken off in the last 40 years in an effort to address large-scale, indeterminate, and multi-level problems.

The focus is on interconnectedness, adaptation, and unpredictability, rather than a mechanistic and reductionist means of science. The method for addressing problems relies on quantitative experimentation through models and simulations, creating computer-assisted or generated versions of real-world scenarios, outcomes, and interventions.

A greater concern with 'anticipatory problems' is also evident. As human geographer Anderson has described: "… Across different domains of life the future is now problematised as a disruption, a surprise. This problematisation of the future as indeterminate or uncertain has been met with an extraordinary proliferation of anticipatory action" (2010, p. 777). He argues that we need to think about the future to avoid assumptions about linear temporality, not as a "… blank separate from the present or that the future is a telos towards which the present is heading" (ibid., p. 778). Similarly, Adams et al. (2009) describe the state of anticipation thinking and living towards the future as a characteristic of our current moment. Anticipation has epistemic value, a virtue emerging through actuarial saturation as sciences of *the actual* are displaced by *speculative forecast.* It is a politics of temporality and affect (2009, p. 246, emphasis in original). Anticipation is commonplace in governing emerging technologies through geo-engineering, nanotechnology, and synthetic biology as soon-to-be problems with still yet unknown social and ethical consequences (Guston, 2010).

As a distinct policy problem category, 'neglected problems' have not been developed fully in the literature, compared with wicked problems and anticipatory problems. The idea of neglect has been considered in the public policy literature but without a name given to it, while the ignorance studies literature has formalised the related concept of ignorance and intensified focus both theoretically and through empirical examples. Bachrach and Baratz in the 1960s already conceptualised the study of governmental decision-making where "Policies reflect not only the preferences and power of those groups whose problems have been addressed" and the ability of groups to limit institutional attention to issues reinforcing or augmenting the status quo (Zahariadis, 2016, p. 2).

A subsequent research interest in what had been understood as the 'pre-political', 'pre-decision-making' and even encompassing non-decision-making in the 1970s, followed in explorations of the 'policy agenda' (Cobb & Elder, 1971). Today, the absence and ignorance sociology literatures open the door to consider further nuances and iterations to how attention, through knowledge and intention, is applied to policy. As a specific policy topic, neglect often encompasses vulnerable groups unable to care adequately for themselves, from children to the elderly who are subjected to a 'passive form of abuse' (Pillemer & Finkelhor, 1988). Still, neglect as a descriptor may have fallen in use over time, as indicated by looking at a Google Books Ngram Viewer (Figure 2.1).

Through these characterisations, there are some general observations to be made. Two states of opposite problem scenarios are commonly described (as shown in Table 2.1). A problem is presumed to be a negative state that is fixed for at least one moment in time, with uncertainty about the state of a problem downplayed, and an imagined possibility of a positive, improved scenario. For the political scientist Nick Turnbull, this direct line is a reliance on the scientific method, to move on an "... artificial, instrumental path from problem to solution" (2008, p. 85).

A name for such a negative-positive scenario is a 'balance routine', used in ignorance studies for the assumption that there are two sides to every problem (Proctor & Schiebinger, 2008). If neglect is a particular problem type, how does a problem come to be identified in the first place? To answer this question, the literature on problematisation and policy problems offers some insights.

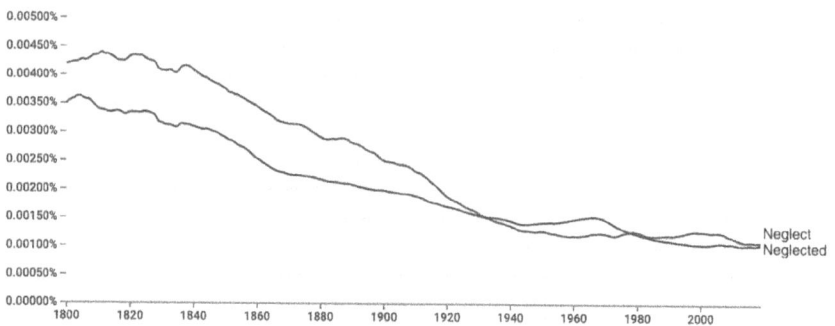

Figure 2.1 References to neglect in books 1800–2019.

(Google Books Ngram Viewer)

Michel Foucault describes problematisation as being about understanding how and why something becomes a problem and the forging of knowledge and relationships to make a certain thing an object of thought (1999). The process of problematisation is not solely a theoretical one. Problematisation, while being a constructed social action, is in fact also "… an 'answer' to a concrete solution which is real" (ibid., p. 75). In relation to science or innovation policy, problematisation has thus been employed to challenge assumptions of a problem in the first place. As Joly notes, problematisation in policy is framed in terms of "… You have a problem and I have the solution" and "… involves the definition of the problem that has to be fixed" (Joly, 2010, p. 6). He gives the example of genetically modified organisms (GMOs) in the 1980s being positioned as a solution for the problem of world hunger and disease, while today the focus has moved onto global warming and sustainable agriculture (ibid).

Such a description of policy problematisation is also the basis of a large literature on framing, as a persistent idea throughout the policy literature (see Daviter, 2007; Lau & Schlesinger, 2005; Steensland, 2008) about how people define and interpret situations or activities, by rendering meaning through the ability to "… locate, perceive, identify, and label" (Goffman, 1974, p. 21). More specifically, framing is the process of constructing a frame, through agency and contention (Benford & Snow, 2000). Frames construct both the problems and possible solutions.

A number of scholars have further researched how 'policy problems' are challenged, by asking what a problem is represented to be within policy (see Gusfield, 1976; Majone, 1989). Carol Bacchi (1999), inspired by Foucault, has further researched problematisation in a policy context to delve into problem conceptualisation in policy by interrogating the assumption that 'problems' are readily identifiable and objective. She reminds us that we mainly mean social problems when discussing problems for policy unique to modern societies (Bacchi, 1999, p. 6).

Social problems tend to be defined as a harmful condition or situation within society. This literature is closely related to policy problem research but with greater emphasis on how society or the public views and constructs problems. For example, Hilgartner and Bosk (1988) in an influential publication highlight the role of public attention in determining the rise and fall of social problems through competition and a need for drama that requires new problem definitions to be repeatedly introduced. Their emphasis is on the public and public arenas, without much consideration of the role of policy, involving other actors and arenas. Chaufan et al. note how the social problem characterisation has fallen out of fashion (2012), perhaps due to the connotation of social problems with moralising, correct and incorrect moral behaviours. It is an explanation for why, in the health arena, social problems have increasingly been reframed as medical problems and can be seen to be part of 'medicalisation' where medical interference oversteps due reason, disguised as care.[2]

Evidence for policy

The push towards treating social or personal problems as technical ones is also reflected in government approaches to policy problems. Governments and policymakers receive a large share of attention in how policy is conceived, what counts as a problem for policy, and the best way to act. Policymakers have been preoccupied with the use of evidence to counter policy being perceived as arbitrary and uninformed, to oppose the claim that "... Policy choices are based on fads, revered exemplars, or abstract theories, rather than solid evidence" (Simmons et al., 2007, p. 451). The use of evidence in policy problematisation has been heavily influenced by the 'evidence-based policy-making' (EBPM) approach, which aims improve policymaking, so that it does not guided by political motivations, laziness or poor practice.[3]

However, the evidence emphasis had been criticised early on in how the approach was projected as one of 'technical, non-partisan problem solvers', while, in fact, they are more akin to lawyers than engineers or scientists, making policy arguments (Majone, 1989). EBPM has also been scrutinised by those who object to "... the continuing influence of the 'modernist' faith in progress informed by reason" (Sanderson, 2002, p. 1) where, as Cairney describes, the roots of EBPM lie in

> ... the early post-war idea that the policymaking process will be improved when we make it more scientific and, therefore, better able to incorporate scientific evidence ... This idea has given way to a more recent sense that policymaking will always be messy, and that an appeal to the primacy of science or 'the evidence' can go too far.
>
> (Cairney, 2015, p. ix)

Evidence can be used in different ways for political means with no guarantee of neutrality and objectivity, which is why some prefer the term 'evidence-influenced' or 'evidence aware' policy (Nutley et al., in Marston & Watts, 2003). A constructivist view may go further to question the existence of an objective scientific knowledge and limits of cultural and historical contingencies when drawing policy implications (Sanderson, 2002, p. 6). On a spectrum of constructivism of 'hard' to 'soft', there are varying degrees of scepticism about scientific knowledge and the relation with social practices (Robbins, 2012). The consequences of a constructivist view are, as Restivo states, that "... problems can be abstracted from their social contexts and solutions sought that do not threaten prevailing social arrangements" (1988, p. 216). He argues that the status quo that produces problems is often left unquestioned through "... social interests, historical and social contexts" (ibid.).

It must also be kept in mind that "... interests, like everything else, can be constructed" (Latour, 2005, p. 145). Interests can inform understandings of actions and behaviour in a policy context, but there is a critique of the 'interest approach' – to be aware of our own constructions in putting forward another representation of the world, and not assume is that interests of actors and their core identities go hand in hand (Webster, 1991, pp. 21–2). Ikeda recognises this fusion of actors and identities in the "... public interest view of public policy, which in effect treats persons who have moved from the private sector to government employment as having been thereby transformed from self-interested profit-seeking actors into public-spirited and selfless public servants" (2002, p. 6). Even differing interests may be constrained by the possible options, as "... policy analysts can appear very similar to policy makers who seek to construct policy problems in ways that match the answers they already have available" (Gale, 2001, p. 384). A bias of which actor holds which interests is important to keep in mind when discussing public health actors.

I have addressed the importance of evidence in producing policy problems as a route to achieve the appearance of technicality, but also relevant is how evidence is presented and what story is told. Policy problems require an outwardly objective and justificational identification corresponding with EBPM to form a narrative of a 'problem state', with clear origins. In this sense, identifying a problem for intervention is often characterised in prescriptive terms of market failure, where market forces or private actors do not provide immediate solutions. For example, WHO director Margaret Chan called for a public–private partnership (PPP) approach to tackling NTDs, in response to market failure of affordable medicines. (WHO, 2013).

Market failure arises from a status quo (or equilibrium) where the market generally provides for societal needs and wants, but when this is not met (e.g. when it is difficult to derive profits or no one is responsible for delivery), government or other non-market actors must amend market conditions or offer provision. NTDs can be understood as a result of market failure for drug and other medical innovations. A typical argument is:

> ... the pharmaceutical industry has little incentive to invest in research and development (R&D) for infectious diseases that predominantly plague poor nations, as medicines cannot be sold there at a price that would allow pharmaceutical firms to cover their high R&D costs.
>
> (Mueller-Langer, 2013, p. 185)

There are aspects missing from such a characterisation. Grounded in welfare economics, market failure is a starting point to summarise a policy and determine future action. In critiquing this economic theory, public choice theorists (interested in economics applied to politics) challenge assumptions of a perfect government rather than focusing on market failure itself (Tullock et al., 2002; Ikeda, 2002). Market failure provides a policy narrative: a starting point and signposting for policy problems, but also directs the potential solution. Another way of challenging a malfunctioning market – or, to that point, a malfunctioning government – is bottom-up, through publics and civil society. One vehicle is through advocacy, particularly social movements, discussed next.

Advocacy through social movements

NTD advocacy involves an element of social movement, as defined by Hess (in Hackett et al., 2008) in a goal of "fundamental social change". This sentiment can be seen in the scientists at the WHO proclaiming: "... it seems to us ethically unacceptable that infected human populations are not administered medication that is freely available while livestock and companion animals are regularly dewormed every year" (Montresor et al., 2013). Scientists have been challenging established organisations from pharma companies and donor countries in their dealing with NTDs, making moral arguments for increased societal concern.

What have scholars said about this type of advocacy? The discussion has tended to centre on social movements, with a focus on state actors such as "science, medicine, and industries", but also patients and other non-state groups (Moore in Hackett et al., 2008, p. 475). Hess also sees scientists as key figures in supporting social movements:

> When scientists step out of their role as researchers to defend the need for policy reform that is contrary to the official articulations of public interest by elites, they form a scientific counterpublic, often in alliance with social movements and other civil society organizations.
>
> (Hess, n.d.)

Scientists can be advocates for policy reform, acting beyond their academic work in establishing projects and organisations, working for NGOs and public institutes; although, when it comes to NTDs, scientists *do not* act predominantly in alliance with social movements and other civil society organisations, as Hess often observes.[4]

Patient action is a gaping hole in policy discussions, and patients are characterised by a minimal political voice, as in this WHO description: "Neglected tropical diseases such as leprosy, lymphatic filariasis and leishmaniasis are feared and the source of strong social stigma and prejudice. As a result, these diseases are often hidden – out of sight, poorly documented and silent" (WHO, 2006, p. 3). It has been scientists who have been central in campaigning for NTD policy change. There is some historical precedence for scientist advocates, as Donohoe notes (2012) in many 'noteworthy examples' of physicians.

One eminent 19th century physician was pathologist Rudolph Virchow, who made valuable contributions to social medicine, arguing many diseases result from the "... unequal distribution of civilization's advantages" (Adams, 1998, p. 339). Thus, he believed physicians to be "... natural advocates of the poor, 'if medicine is really to accomplish its great task it must intervene in political and social life' ..." (Virchow quoted in Adams, 1998, p. 339). Virchow was an advocate through his socially minded philosophical views and voicing his opinion against child labour, and for public medical care, universal education, and democracy (ibid.). This move is what made him an archetype of the politically engaged medical scientist. For Adams, ironically the leading scientist was deemed a radical in his commitment to the idea that (medical) science was also political, and view that only under certain political circumstances could scientific truth be made apparent (1998, p. 160).

In the history of tropical medicine, it has also been a precarious position to be a policy-engaged scientist. Worboys notes that Sir Patrick Manson, often called the 'father of tropical medicine' through his public reputation, was appointed physician and medical advisor to the Colonial Office in 1897 (in Lemaine et al., 1976, p. 85). He acted in the capacity of a 'firm's doctor' in an 'influential policy-advisory role' with direct access to the Secretary of State (ibid.). However, this position was officially mandated and compared starkly with his contemporary Ronald Ross, who, as a working scientist, was firmly rebuked in his suggestion to the Colonial Office of a new scheme of sanitary commissioners. Lemaine et al. saw the message as "... scientists should confine themselves to research and not become involved in practical policy" (ibid., p. 92). Scientists could be instrumental in policy, but there was a small scope in how to do so, only if formally designated, with limited room for influence.

In other circumstances, it is evident that science and politics cannot be easily separated. The book 'Doctors for Democracy', about the 1990 Nepali revolution and instigated by a group of medical professionals, illustrates this point well: "Observing that social inequality and poverty were the root causes of ill health among the masses, some doctors reasoned that the most direct medical interventions they could promote were those of political and social reform" (Adams, 1998, pp. 4–5). The rationalisation of the role of politics in science reflects a desire for scientific fact to be independent of society and politics.

A view is that politics may compromise objectivity but the example of the Nepalese doctors showed that:

> Politics, in their view, could be used to reveal and attend to objective truths and therefore could enhance medical practice without comprom- ising scientific objectivity. This objectivity was born from the perceived efficacy of technical interventions provided by a scientific approach to social problems.
>
> (ibid.)

Adams argues that medicine differs as a socially engaged humanistic science as opposed to pure science, with the politicisation of medicine through pol- itically active medical professionals merging two insights: "(1) that medicine must become political to eradicate the cause of ill health and (2) that med- ically scientific truths are usually formulated in contested political contexts" (ibid., p. 172).

Scientists, in seeking to address problems in health through activism, challenge the politics-science distinction. Next, I turn to innovation, as presented as a solution to policy problems, to explore the underlining theor- etical frameworks employed to understand how NTDs are addressed.

Innovation conceptualisation for solutions

Science has long been presented as a solution to societal problems. The 20th century saw the transformative effect of 'big science' on society through a 'leap in scale and organisation', with physics and chemistry becoming dir- ectly useful, goal-directed economic endeavour (Riecken, 1969). Some, such as Riecken, have argued that science has more implications for 'action' than social sciences (ibid.), and, similarly, Turnbull sees science as a 'sophisticated expression' of problem-solving rationality (2008, pp. 82–4).

Innovation poses a new relationship with policy problems. In a conven- tional and widespread definition of "… bringing a new product into the market or into practical use" (Schroeder, 2007, p. 37), the emphasis is on eco- nomic significance. Therefore, innovation connects science and technology to the economy and it is also viewed as intrinsically positive and desirable (Webster, 1991, p. 35). Innovation is presented as a solution to many of the challenges faced on big global topics such as health, the environment, pov- erty, and well-being.

The main measure of the level of innovation is through research and development (R&D) but measuring the impact of policies related to science, technology, and innovation has faced difficulties; and the statistical relationship between economic growth and R&D investment has not proved very forthcoming (Webster, 1991, p. 100).[5] R&D investment forms part of a linear model of innovation. Godin points out: "One of the first (theoretical) frameworks developed for historically understanding the relation of science and technology to the economy has been the 'linear model of innovation' ..." (2006, p. 639). The model describes the process of technological change sequentially from an idea (drawing from the science base through basic research then applied research) that moves to development, production, and finally diffusion within markets and wider society.[6] As a model, it outlines a linear progression of discrete stages, shown in the Figure 2.2 below.

The model is linear because it is based on an input-output framework that progresses from one stage to another through a series of steps. For NTDs, the assumption is that an input change will result in outputs that mean these diseases are better dealt with.[7] The demand-pull model was an early alternative to the linear model, providing a supply-side view of innovation.[8] The supply-side view posits that investment in R&D and scientific discovery leads to innovation, while the demand side comes from the opposite direction in that consumers drive innovation through market demand. The linear model of innovation is widely adopted, in making this relationship between R&D, innovation, and economic growth (despite critique of the model as not reflecting complexity and collaborative or more open ways of doing innovation).

A similar reversal in the demand-pull to supply-push example of linearity can be found in the relationship between health, innovation, and development. The idea of 'development for health' has long been established. A first point is that poverty and low socio-economic status causes ill health, shown by the political economy of health (Doyal & Pennell, 1979) and social determinants of health (SDH) literatures (Marmot, 2007). A second point, applied to a country level, is that the economy needs to develop first for health outcomes to improve. This argument comes from a technocratic interpretation of 'stages of development' where economic development is sought first with societal improvement expected to follow. Countries want to move up the escalator of progress

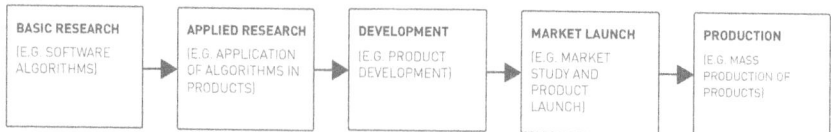

Figure 2.2 'The linear model of innovation'.

(Bhirud, Rodrigues, & Desai, 2005)

through 'Rostow's stages theory' of economic growth "... from a pre-industrial state to full economic maturity" (see Rostow, 1971). This 'stages theory' was prevalent in the early post-war period – with the idea of moving across innovation in agricultural, to manufacturing, to industrial and commercial sections – where to miss a stage could be a disaster:

> ... development proceeds through a linear succession of stages copied from the historical experience of existing industrial countries. This was a historicism in drawing theory from past experiences or examples but also wanted to do away with connections to the past that do not match a pursuit of modernity ...
>
> (Biel, 2000, p. 74)

The idea would later be reversed, such that health could precede and contribute to development. As Morel describes: "Health, science and technology are increasingly being recognised as prerequisites for economic and social development, and not merely as their consequences" (2003, p. S35). Linearity is reversed from 'development to health' to 'health for development' (see Figure 2.3, below), and this change had important implications for global health policy. Instead of identifying poor health being caused by underdevelopment, improved health is a reason leading to economic development, as a marker of a country's progress, understood through common metrics to measure improvements in a country (e.g. GDP, literacy, life expectancy, poverty rates). Policies addressing health then moves away from a systemic emphasis to economic development (on policies and investment in health systems and infrastructure) to vertical programmes addressing individual health issues.

Development for health

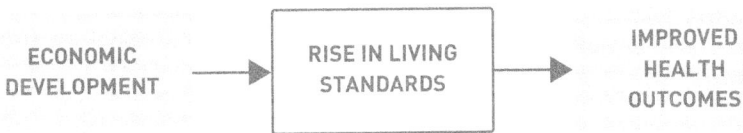

Health for Development

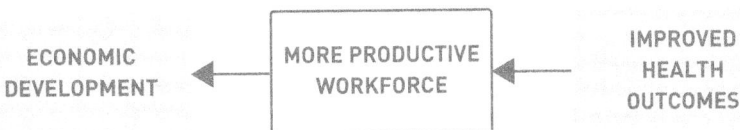

Figure 2.3 Reverse linearity of development for health.

The switch in emphasis to 'health for development' can be seen in the policy arguments for NTDs as diseases said to be both a cause and result of poverty and underdevelopment, in a self-reinforcing cycle, with health accepted as a precursor. As a result, demonstrating impact upon economic development reinforces the rationale for intervention in NTDs.

China was shown to be proof, through the so-called barefoot doctors, that it was economically advantageous to invest in health, but that could also be achieved through social innovation rather than only scientific or techno-logical innovation (Zhang et al., 2008). China's community health workers, nicknamed barefoot doctors, had elementary training in diagnostics, immun-isation, education, simple treatment, and liaised with the qualified medical sector. They were a cheap resource to improve health and a politically driven health intervention being used to promote economic development. Adams (1998), in exploring the linking of politics and medicine, gives the example of the barefoot doctor programme to reflect the "... call for political solutions to basic health problems" (pp. 166–7). The programme was seen by many as a successful intervention, driven by supportive political ideals of the Cultural Revolution in 1966 to reject high technology, such that, "... basic essentials of scientific medical intervention were recast in a framework that made national medical traditions appropriate for health care in the Chinese countryside" (ibid., p. 167). 'Expert' knowledge was seen to be opposed to 'Red' knowledge and thus downgraded. Also discredited to an extent were the stages of devel-opment in which 'development for health' was grounded.

A move towards the 'health for development' model allows NTDs to be more appealing as a concern and has shaped the means of dealing with these diseases. Similar to the example of barefoot doctors, the shift to 'health for development' is grounded in a view of the type of expertise that can provide legitimate evidence. Therefore, expert knowledge being relied upon becomes central to determining how policy problems and solutions are viewed. I take this consideration of expertise further in the next section, which deals with the various disciplinary lenses that have been applied to NTDs.

Disciplinary influences

From discussing the literature relating to problematisation and engaged with solutions proposed through innovation and the role of models, next, I develop further the idea of how disciplines guide policy problem-solving by exploring the expertise of economics, history, and an interdisciplinary lens, including anthropology and epidemiology. What one discipline offers to policy over others depends on a number of factors.

Economic thinking is prevalent throughout approaches to policy problems and in policymaking because economic impact is both desirable and a marker of progress, with a perception that the economics discipline is able to foresee and influence such outcomes. According to McCloskey (1998), a chief goal of economics is prediction and control, but other disciplinary approaches may be downplayed; and economics is sometimes accused of ignoring other political and social considerations.

Majone (1989) also posited that the very methodology of policymaking – 'decisionism' – favours economics as a generalised logic of choice, where political actors make rational choices from available alternatives, as the best means to achieve objectives. Here, subdisciplines, microeconomics and decision theory have been influential, with policy analysts seeking to extend principles of rational choice from private economic transactions to public policymaking. Policy approaches based on rational decision-makers may now be outmoded, but their legacy can be found as a product of bringing behavioural economics into policymaking, assuming irrational rather than rational actors (Thaler & Sunstein, 2008). Economic approaches and ideas prevailing in policy are described as 'economicisation' (or 'economisation'), where "…an aspect of practices, procedures and activities in which the calculability of things is put forward and in which, accordingly, action is subjected to optimality and hence made prone to economic assessment" (Muniesa & Linhardt, 2009, p. 12). For NTDs, a focus on economic rationale for policies is example of economicisation.

Another disciplinary approach I address is history. Historicism has still been a popular current in policy theories and prescriptions, present, for example, in the stages of economic growth theory. A definitionally vague and broad term, Karl Popper defined historicism as predicting the future course of history and thought it to be a poor method because the growth of knowledge produces uncertainty in the future such that it is impossible to be predictive based on the past (1957). However, as Reynolds (2008) discusses, the alternative meaning of 'mundane historicism' is more than the predicting tool of Popper. With roots in opposition to the enlightenment ideal of an ahistorical and universal rationality, mundane historicism uses historical context. Also, 'methodological historicism' understands history as distinct from natural sciences, and 'Popperian historicism' in predictive power to find laws, rhythms, and patterns in history (ibid.).

History, both mundane and methodological, to inform policymaking and better understand public policy has had some resurgence (see Berridge, 2008; Guldi & Armitage, 2014; Rennie, 1998).[9] This may be a lighter version of historicism in using historical fact to 'confirm' theory, interpretation, and even prediction. Historicism in the non-Popperian, mundane sense provides the content to theories of knowledge and, for NTDs, has been a defining feature of theories of science, innovation, and economic development applied to disease.

Historiography is perhaps more straightforward to define as a methodology, in the study of the history of historical writing, how individual historians have interpreted events and, by extension, historical work on a specific topic (such as tropical diseases). The historiography of tropical diseases and tropical medicine is an ongoing project, ordered through national institutions, scientists, perspectives, and transnational networks of colony or empire. One aspect of this historiography, then, has been the focus on the "… conventional portrayal of tropical medicine" as being "… imbedded in the imperial enterprise of their respective countries", while the colonised context adds "neocolonial, developmentalist, nationalist, and patriotic features to tropical medicine" (Coutinho in Armus, 2003, p. 90). Coutinho argues that an endemic disease became a problem to the coloniser when the colony was theirs and once independence was gained, the disease became part of the newly independent country's search for national identity. Therefore, a consideration of historicism informing policy runs throughout this book, although it is the historiography of tropical medicine and tropical diseases that forms a basis for charting the policy development of NTDs.

Historians and economists, to whom I will add epidemiologists and anthropologists, all have growing positions within global health policy, often as part of interdisciplinary teams. More interdisciplinary work is happening through the integration of societal issues and concerns into scientific practice. Although Doubleday and Viseu (2010) have questioned the lack of significant discussion on the inclusion of social science, they are wary that "… policy documents suggest this integration is a relatively straightforward process" (ibid., p. 55). One solution offered has been to standardise and manage interdisciplinary work through a close working relationship with research subjects, including a sometimes contributory or collaboratory role to their research or an attempt to somehow change, inform, or add to existing practices that are related. This 'embedded research' is not a neutral position, with the implications discussed in the remainder of this section.

Parker, Polman, and Allen (2016, p. S6) note how, in the context of NTDs, scholars of different disciplines have worked collaboratively. Most commonly, if they were more senior, they would work separately on their own research, though in 'parallel tramlines', or as 'handmaidens of biomedicine' if more junior in schools of public health:

> … In the world of NTDs, and global health more generally, it would be fair to say that it is rare indeed for an epidemiologist, parasitologist or public health specialist to work on an equal footing with an anthropologist, historian or political scientist.
>
> (Parker, Polman, & Allen, 2016, p. S6)

They describe the 'qualitative' social research that is undertaken as elaborating on a "… 'factorial model of disease' with complex social and cultural processes being conceptualised as discrete, measurable 'factors', acting as 'barriers' to the effective implementation of global health interventions" (ibid.).

This is a relatively critical perspective taken by Parker and Allen, who are anthropologists (Polman is an epidemiologist). Anthropologists have been sought after in public health and biomedical research to unlock 'cultural secrets' in being able to understand and gather insight from local communities (Krumeich, et al., 2001). In turn, they have also found in health a rich topic of research, hence the emergence of the 'medical anthropologist' in the 1960s (Basehart, 1964) and also the prominent examples of researchers with training in both medicine and anthropology (e.g. Farmer et al., 2006; Farmer et al., 2013). Writer Robert Desowitz noticed this changing positioning of anthropologists:

> The generic anthropologist began to disappear in the 1950s and 1960s. The biomedical researchers–geneticists, epidemiologists, and microbiologists discovered the anthropologist's utility in gaining entry into tribal groups as well as their providing a ready-made source of important demographic data. In turn, the anthropologists discovered biology and their calling evolved into specialities.
>
> (2004, p. 178)

For anthropological research on NTDs, the focus is often on aetiology, signs or symptoms, treatments, and experiences of individual diseases.[10] Anthropologists Parker and Allen are among the few who have looked at NTDs as a group, although they do so by country and are interested in the control method for five of the NTDs called 'mass drug administration' (MDA), which Allen describes as "… the largest global health programme that the world has ever seen" (2013).

They are interested in advocacy for NTDs and have been critical of aspects, including what they see as an over-promise in the global drive for NTDs, through 'grand claims' and aspirations to achieve the 'Millennium Development Goals' (MDGs) and 'making poverty history'. In their view, NTD aspirations have generated unprecedented attention to NTDs (Parker & Allen, 2011, p. 2). Through a community study in Uganda, they ask the question: "Does mass drug administration for the integrated treatment of neglected tropical diseases really work?" (2011). Again, the question of politicisation returns as a concern:

> Large amounts of funding are being allocated to the control of neglected tropical diseases. Strategies primarily rely on the mass distribution of drugs to adults and children living in endemic areas. The approach is presented as morally appropriate, technically effective, and context-free.
>
> (2013, p. 224)

As Adams describes, postmodern critical theory politicises social problems "… by situating them in historical and cultural contexts, to implicate themselves in the process of collecting and analyzing data, and to relativize their findings" (Lindlof & Taylor, 2011, p. 52). The charge of Parker and Allen is that, "… normative ideas about global health programs are used to set aside social and biological evidence" (ibid.). As anthropologists, it is the 'local details' that are set aside, but also the country context:

> ... resistance to the take-up of free drugs was linked by many of those with whom we lived to a sense of marginalization, and sometimes outright oppression by the Ugandan government ... while some people benefitted from the treatment program, it was unrealistic to assume that it would lift such impoverished and politically excluded populations out of poverty. It is mostly neglected people who are infected with neglected diseases – and this fact could not just be wished away.
>
> (ibid., p. 224)

In '(D)e-politicizing parasites: reflections on attempts to control the control of neglected tropical diseases', Parker and Allen use Ferguson's 'antipolitics' thesis (1994) as a starting point. The original critique by Ferguson related to the aid and development industry, arguing that social realities were depoliticised as a way of giving control, and technical solutions implemented context-free using international expertise. Parker and Allen view his account as ignoring the complexities of the development industry and find it more interesting how rhetoric was believed, such that the depoliticisation discourse was used as a tool to promote vested interests.

Parker and Allen employ a depoliticisation argument for their own research, directed at the scientists, policymakers, and development workers implementing NTD policies. They challenge how the optimism for MDA in controlling NTDs, driven by these actors, ignores a political view of intervention acceptance and whether it was dealing with the root problem. What does not come across so clearly was that Parker and Allen were invited by one of the scientists they are indirectly critical of – Alan Fenwick – who runs the Schistosomiasis Control Initiative (SCI), and who enabled them to be embedded in the project to implement MDA in Uganda (Reisz, 2013). As described in a *Times* newspaper article in 2013 they carried out their research: "in close collaboration with [those responsible for the control of the worms, insects or snails that transmit diseases], and with relevant district authorities" (ibid.). Opposition between disciplines came out in their research through an apparent contradiction between an anthropological outlook and the advocacy work of scientists and other actors.

Perhaps less-contentious interdisciplinary working can be said to be in the emergence of interdisciplinary fields, where the convergence of academic fields is a process of compromise. 'Health economics' is thought to have begun in the 1960s through work on markets for healthcare and models of health production to account for demand in health (Cardoso, 2008). Since then, economists[11] have gained a greater role in public health, leading to the wide adoption of concepts and tools such as the 'Global Burden of Disease' work, and development of the 'disability-adjusted life year' (DALY) measure[12] by the health economist Chris Murray with epidemiologist Alan Lopez. Next I take a broader view of global health policy as a field and focus on the particular policy landscape for NTDs.

Global health actors and landscape

To understand NTDs as a policy problem also involves a discussion on how global health contributes to the constitution of policy problems. Global health policies did not come into being until after 'global' institutions such as the WHO were established in the 1950s (Brown et al., 2006; Ng & Ruger, 2011; Ruger, 2005). Tropical diseases and now 'neglected' tropical diseases straddle these two eras of public health spanning the health exploits of empire and colonialisation. The first directions of efforts were mainly to benefit the colonisers, with the colonised as second priority (Trouiller et al., 2002), and the problems of disease were sometimes worsened by colonisers (Farley, 2003, p. 2).[13] Post-empire priorities were similarly skewed. In the dying days of empire, the 'triumph' of tropical medicine was the "… last justification for imperialism" (ibid.) and after colonies gained independence, 'health of the natives' was used as a justification for ongoing colonial presence (e.g. the continuation of the US military in the Philippines and Puerto Rico) (Biss, 2014).

'Global' health now means that, theoretically, the health of the poorest populations is prioritised. The idea of 'public' health, whether on a national level or globally, is meant to be for everyone; but what it really means is for the poor (Biss, 2014). The rich can already guarantee health to a large extent, so to make health 'public' is to enable access and quality of care for those who cannot easily pay. On a country level, making health public extends from health systems and basic infrastructure to trained medical practitioners and researchers. There is still some debate about the difference between global health and public health, but a number of scholars argue they are not usefully distinguishable today.[14]

How did global health emerge, and what is its difference to international health? International health has generally referred to epidemics spanning across geographical borders. The internationalisation of public health resulted in a demarcation of tropical diseases from development. Kelly and Beisel (2011) summarise the changes:

> On one hand, the creation of the WHO as distinct from agencies such as the International Monetary Fund narrowed the scope of public health initiatives. On the other, the internationalization of public health and the subsequent dismantling of colonial governments centralized medical expertise; health decisions were no longer the province of local governments but of committees in Geneva and New York.
>
> (Kelly & Beisel, 2011, p. 76)

Global health is concerned with the public health needs of all people, regardless of national boundaries (Brown et al., 2006). If this is the ideal strived for, international health becomes outmoded. As Harman (2014) notes, during the West African Ebola epidemic (2013–5), the response was "… indicative of international rather than global health governance" in the failure of co-operation and collaboration, which did not happen across institutions and states.

The institutional set-up changed from a local to global system of economic governance following World War II, including medical research towards 'large-scale science' that is "… driven by public-private partnerships, international research collaborations and large-scale development donors" (Schumaker in Cooter & Pickstone, 2003, p. 78). Looking at trends of data on global funding towards public health indicates where economic governance is being driven. In 1990, global health funding was dominated by the WHO alongside USA and other donor countries including France, Sweden, and Japan – but by 2010, the NGO share had increased dramatically, particularly from new funds (IHME, 2010). These included 'The Global Fund to Fight AIDS, Tuberculosis and Malaria' (GFATM), the Global Alliance for Vaccines and Immunization (GAVI) and the Bill and Melinda Gates Foundation (ibid.). Funding for NTDs has followed a similar pattern, except industry funding plays a bigger role, which is most likely to be due to the drug solution focus.

The 'Global Funding of Innovation for Neglected Diseases (G-FINDER) Survey' has been tracking funding patterns for investment in NTDs (Policy Cures Research, 2020). While the tracking only covers R&D, it is capturing some wider trends. Public investment is still the biggest funding source, but is followed by the private sector and philanthropic organisations, with industry investment increasing 'dramatically' (ibid.). The increase reflects how, over the past decade, the multinational pharmaceutical companies – so-called 'big pharma' – made concerted efforts to engage with certain global health issues, and have been drawn to NTDs in recent years.

Therefore, global health has emerged from an institutionalisation and globalising of health, which has seen the entrance of new, predominately private sector and philanthropic health actors. Critical global health researchers have focused on new health actors but also the response and changing role of the WHO since its creation (Biehl & Petryna, 2013; McInnes et al., 2012). The WHO, with some variability, has remained a central player with strategic influence, including for NTDs, involved with framing the policy problem and not straying far from the first 2006 report on NTDs description:

> With little political voice, neglected tropical diseases have a low profile and status in public health priorities. Lack of reliable statistics and

unpronounceable names of diseases have all hampered efforts to bring
them out of the shadows.

(WHO, 2006, p. II)

To conclude this chapter, I turn to understandings of neglect that go beyond
those of the established institutions such as the WHO.

Conclusion: neglect as a policy characterisation

Returning to the types of problem characterisations, neglect has a unique
link with health, as the absence of concern or care, with care being central
to public health, from a micro level of caring for the sick to the macro of
caring for populations and caring about what makes them sick.[15] Conversely,
Sophie Harman (2012), in looking at care in global health governance, finds
that different practices of policy can promote care and, in some cases, the
opposite – harm, which is why she describes 'neglected health' as a result
of the dominance of one issue over another. Neglected health, happens in
issues "… sidelined or ignored because of global prioritising" (ibid., p. 122).
It means that the success advocacy of some, for example, pandemic and
emerging disease fears (HIV/AIDS, pandemic flu, Ebola, now COVID-19)
has a negative effect on others. Therefore, care applied disproportionately,
or too much care directed to certain issues, can produce neglect. But how is
care decided upon and, normatively, why do we care about some issues over
others?

Caring for NTDs happens in a different way to other health issues. Situating
NTDs as the 'other' has an effect in how they are imagined as diseases. The
imagination of neglect is explored in the absence literature, as Balmer and
Rappert (2016) put it, topics generate concern or 'non-concern' and take the
limelight, setting priorities and policy agendas. Rappert highlights how it is
in the 'social problem' and 'social movement' literatures, where there is an
implicit commentary, that those matters do not generate interest and debate.
An imaginary of neglect is thus present in thinking about why topics are in
the limelight, and also how priority- and agenda-setting decisions are made.
Absence theorists are interested in why there is lack of concern, interest, and
debate for topics, and why we think some topics matter and others not – it is
not spelt out, but this is neglect.

Similarly, the call to action by the ignorance studies literature resonates with
understanding the nature of neglect. As Proctor and Schiebinger describe, in
their seminal book in the field, 'Agnotology: The Making and Unmaking of
Ignorance', neglect is a mechanism behind ignorance:[16]

… Our goal here is to explore how ignorance is produced or maintained
in diverse settings, through mechanisms such as deliberate or inadvertent

neglect, secrecy and suppression, document destruction, unquestioned tradition, and myriad forms of inherent (or avoidable) culturopolitical selectivity.

(2008, pp. vii–viii)

Therefore, deliberate or inadvertent neglect is the act that produces or
maintains ignorance. The distinction of intention implies it can be done consciously or not, as a purposeful lack of concern or care, or even inadvertent
or systematic. It may be inadvertent neglect through misunderstanding or
because inquiry is selective or out of necessity. Going one step further, deliberate ignorance can be caused by neglect that is actively engineered and used
as a strategic ploy to control social processes. This tactical component means
that ignorance may be politicised, and directs focus towards who is creating
ignorance and why. Proctor and Schiebinger go on to state the connection
with forms of knowledge as a reason for neglect:

Our primary purpose here is to promote the study of ignorance, by
developing tools for understanding how and why various forms of knowledge have 'not come to be' or disappeared, or have been delayed or long
neglected, for better or for worse, at various points in history.

(ibid.)

There is a role in highlighting neglect, as Abeysinghe the claims to ignorance or
neglect "… can sometimes serve to promote policy production" (Abeysinghe,
2015). To highlight neglect is important, in how issues are identified or not,
and how they are formulated as problems for redress through institutions and
their mitigation procedures. As Proctor and Schiebinger (2008) put it, things
are not simply present and absent – they are made so, in what is concealed
and revealed or whether it is an issue of concern or non-concern (ibid., p. 6).
Interestingly, neglect appears to be an important characterisation of ignorance as a research problem, "… this strategy can also lead to an acknowledgement of non-knowledge that so far has been neglected, but is suddenly taken
seriously and may even be seen as fundamental" (Gross, 2007, p. 748).

The neglect of non-knowledge is a feature of why ignorance has not been
researched extensively in the past, as "… closed ignorance means that 'we
either neglect problems themselves, or do not take notice of intuitive insights,
experience, information, models and methods of solution which are available
inside of society'…" (ibid.). This is a presentation of ignorance as a field of
study that has not been given due attention – it has been neglected and deserves
a concerted effort to rectify. However, neglect itself is a different characterisation to absence or ignorance in the implicit assignment of blame and responsibility, and an unequal relationship between the neglector and the neglected.
Crucially, what needs attention is not simply this or that missing recognition.
The type of absence becomes a central point to understand, as neglect is a special type of absence – the object of neglect in NTDs is defined by what it is not.

This chapter has demonstrated how the literature on policy problems and solutions is closely tied to questions about the use of evidence and advocacy in policy, as well as the disciplinary lens through which to view problem-solving. However, it is the ignorance literature that offers alternative views of knowledge to help to explain the structural and directed causes of neglect. These strands of policy dialogue will be connected again in the proceeding chapters, in how policy problems are prioritised or not, imagined to be neglected, and subject to advocacy and profiling. Global health policy has become an active field with numerous new actors and disciplinary contributors. The connections and divisions in an evolving global health landscape, and in understanding neglect, will be further examined. The empirical research will uncover the various events and milestones that have made up the recent policy history of NTDs. Next, I delve into the case of NTDs as a policy problem, analysing the conceptual origins and what the dominant strategies for tackling these diseases have been, and why.

Notes

1   In 'problem types', I mean ideal types in the Weberian sense as an abstract, hypothetical concept (Hekman, 1983) to produce a broad characterisation of the nature of a problem.

2   Ivan Illich (1975) argues how the wide definition of ill health expands the scope of medical care, the outcome of which is a denial of humanity in the process of "… transforming pain, illness, and death from a personal problem into a technical [one]" (Illich, 2003 in Chaufan et al., 2012). He used the 'Pyrrhic victories over some tropical diseases' as an example of the belief in an almost limitless progress of medicine, which would then face new challenges in the perpetuation of disease through economic and technological factors (1975, p. 73).

3   According to Ian Sanderson, EBPM is derived from 'evidence-based medicine' (EBM) in seeking to use information and knowledge more effectively to justify intervention, particularly in the UK and US (2002).

4   Related developments have been the 'political opportunity structure' literature developed by sociologists to look at the conditions where social movements influence policy structures, as well as the 'advocacy coalition framework' in public policy to look at the influence of competing interest groups on policy outcomes (Sell & Prakash, 2004, p. 146). Similarly, Frickel and Gross argue scientific and intellectual movements or 'SIMs' as "collective efforts to pursue research programs or projects for thought in the face of resistance from others in the scientific or intellectual community" (Frickel & Gross, 2005, p. 206).

5   Martin and Scott in surveying the related literature summarise in these terms: "the level of investment in research and development is likely to be too low, from a social point of view, whether market structure is nearly atomistic, a highly concentrated oligopoly, or something in between" (2000, p. 438). What counts as R&D is also a point of contention – with companies stretching the concept of R&D to claim tax benefits.

6 Godin also notes two further generations of the linear model – a statistical correlation between research and economic growth, productivity, industrial competitiveness, and 'National Innovation Systems' (NIS). Adoption of the linear model has fed into a larger policy project justifying government support of science and innovation, as well as the role of "industrialists, consultants and business schools, seconded by economists" in a theoretical construction of innovation (Godin, 2006, pp. 640–1).

7 Godin argues that the linear model never existed in the form and usage depicted by later theorists arguing for an abandonment of the model in favour of a new version (Grandin, Wormbs, & Widmalm, 2004; Godin & Lane, 2013).

8 Also, Keynesian economics, widely accepted post-war up until the 1970s and encouraged the consideration of demand-side factors.

9 Haddon et al., who asked policymakers about the value of history, found history was viewed as a source of knowledge about a policy area, providing instructive parallels, challenging existing paradigms and identifying paradigm shifts (2015).

10 For example, anthropologists have uncovered reasons for low take-up of drugs because of the experience of schistosomiasis differing for children and adults (Hewlett & Cline, 1997). Many may be asymptomatic, but blood in the urine making 'red urine' only tends to be a sign of infection in children, so there is a perception that adults do not suffer from the same infection. Adults, then, are more reluctant to take drugs.

11 For a sociological review of the health economist, see (Ashmore, Mulkay, & Pinch, 1989).

12 Described as a "... systematic effort to quantify the comparative magnitude of health loss due to diseases, injuries, and risk factors by age, sex, and geography over time" (IHME, http://healthdata.org, accessed 2/4/14).

13 For example, the 'scorched earth' policies of clearing land, and insecticide used to control rinderpest in cattle, exacerbated sleeping sickness in human populations (Scoones, 2014).

14 Public health may have the furthest historical roots in the "sanitary movement and contagion eras" (Awofeso, 2004, p. 705). Both encompass a population-based health study to view health as a problem of populations and not only on an individual or group basis. This population perspective has grown in popularity alongside epidemiology and health economics to look at causes and understandings of health beyond strict biomedical determination. Fried et al. argue: "Global health and public health are indistinguishable. Both view health in terms of physical, mental, and social wellbeing, rather than merely the absence of disease. Both emphasise population-level policies, as well as individual approaches to health promotion. And both address the root causes of ill-health through a broad array of scientific, social, cultural, and economic strategies" (Fried et al., 2010, p. 535).

15 Chaufan et al. (2012) see a tension between 'cure' and 'care', reflected in the historic preference of the US government to invest in NIH biomedical research budgets over basic access or universal healthcare. This may be taken to be illustrative also of the innovation approaches discussed as a response against neglect that relies on feeling and thought, rather than action and information.

16 Agnotology refers to "... the study of culturally induced uncertainty" (Stilgoe, 2016).

References

Abeysinghe, S. 2015. "Ignorance Claims as a Call to Action: The Case of Neglected Tropical Diseases." Accessed March 29, 2016. https://icpublicpolicy.org/conference/file/reponse/1433940937.pdf.

Adams, V. 1998. *Doctors for Democracy: Health Professionals in the Nepal Revolution.* Cambridge University Press. https://books.google.com/books?id=x1sH6FrnpVYC&pgis=1.

Adams, V., Murphy, M., & Clarke, A. E. 2009. "Anticipation: Technoscience, Life, Affect, Temporality." *Subjectivity* 28 (1): 246–65. https://doi.org/10.1057/sub.2009.18

Allen, T. 2016. Deworming Delusions: Mass Treatment for African Parasites in a Biosocial Perspective. *Journal of Biosocial Science.* 2016 Sep; 48 Suppl 1: S116–47. doi: 10.1017/S0021932016000171. PMID: 27428063.

Anderson, B. 2010. "Preemption, Precaution, Preparedness: Anticipatory Action and Future Geographies." *Progress in Human Geography* 34 (6): 777–98. https://doi.org/10.1177/0309132510362600.

Armus, D. 2003. *Disease in the History of Modern Latin America: From Malaria to AIDS.* Duke University Press.

Ashmore, M., Mulkay, M. J., & Pinch, T. 1989. *Health and Efficiency: A Sociology of Health Economics.* Open University Press.

Awofeso, N. 2004. "What's New about the 'New Public Health'?" *American Journal of Public Health* 94 (5): 705–9. https://ncbi.nlm.nih.gov/pubmed/15117684.

Bacchi, C. L. 1999. *Women, Policy and Politics.* Sage.

Basehart, H. W. 1964. "Biennial Review of Anthropology 1963." *The Americas* 21 (01): 103–5. https://doi.org/10.2307/979722.

Benford, R. D., & Snow, D. A. 2000. "Framing Processes and Social Movements: An Overview and Assessment." *Annual Review of Sociology* 26 (1): 611–39. https://doi.org/10.1146/annurev.soc.26.1.611.

Berridge, V. 2008. "History Matters? History's Role in Health Policy Making." *Medical History* 52 (3): 311–26. https://pubmedcentral.nih.gov/articlerender.fcgi?artid=2448976&tool=pmcentrez&rendertype=abstract.

Bhirud, S., Rodrigues, L., & Desai, P. 2005. "Knowledge Sharing Practices in Km: A Case Study in Indian Software Subsidiary." *Journal of Knowledge Management Practice.* https://google.co.uk/search?q=Knowledge+Sharing+Practices+In+Km:A+Case+Study+In+Indian+Software+Subsidiary&ie=utf-8&oe=utf-8&gws_rd=cr&ei=UIRWWP7nIYvpwAKKupHACQ.

Biehl, J., & Petryna, A. 2013. *When People Come First: Critical Studies in Global Health.* Princeton University Press.

Biel, R. 2000. *The New Imperialism: Crisis and Contradictions in North–South Relations.* Zed Books. https://books.google.co.uk/books/about/The_New_Imperialism.html?id=u1C3AAAAIAAJ&pgis=1.

Bill & Melinda Gates Foundation. n.d. "Grand Challenges." http://gcgh.grandchallenges.org/.

Biss, E. 2014. *On Immunity: An Inoculation.* Graywolf Press.

Brown, T. M., Cueto, M., & Fee, E. 2006. "The World Health Organization and the Transition from 'International' to 'Global' Public Health." *American Journal of Public Health* 96 (1): 62–72. https://doi.org/10.2105/AJPH.2004.050831.

Cairney, P. 2012. "Complexity Theory in Political Science and Public Policy." *Political Studies Review* 10 (3): 346–58. https://doi.org/10.1111/j.1478-9302.2012.00270.x.

Cairney, P. 2015. *The Politics of Evidence-Based Policy Making.* Springer.

Cardoso, C. 2008. "Health Economics or Health Care Economics?" *Tékhne - Revista de Estudos Politécnicos* (10): 189–98.

Chaufan, C., Hollister, B., Nazareno, J., & Fox, P. 2012. "Medical Ideology as a Double-Edged Sword: The Politics of Cure and Care in the Making of Alzheimer's Disease." *Social Science & Medicine* 74 (5): 788–95. https://doi.org/10.1016/j.socscimed.2011.10.033.

Cobb, R. W., & Elder, C. D. 1971. "The Politics of Agenda-Building: An Alternative Perspective for Modern Democratic Theory." *The Journal of Politics* 33 (4): 892–915. https://doi.org/10.2307/2128415.

Cooter, R., & Pickstone, J. V. 2003. *Companion to Medicine in the Twentieth Century.* Taylor & Francis.

Daviter, F. 2007. "Policy Framing in the European Union." *Journal of European Public Policy* 14 (4): 654–66. https://doi.org/10.1080/13501760701314474.

Desowitz, R. S. 2004. *Federal Bodysnatchers and the New Guinea Virus: People, Parasites, Politics.* W. W. Norton & Company. https://books.google.co.uk/books/about/Federal_Bodysnatchers_and_the_New_Guinea.html?id=s37APnXo2zQC&pgis=1.

Donohoe, M. 2012. *Public Health and Social Justice.* John Wiley. https://books.google.com/books?id=2cuCvmSTlrkC&pgis=1.

Doubleday, R., & Viseu, A. 2010. *Questioning Interdisciplinarity: What Roles for Laboratory based Social Science in Nano Meets Macro: Social Perspectives on Nanoscale Sciences and Technologies.* Edited by K. Kjolberg & F. E. Wickson. Pan Stanford Publishing. https://books.google.com/books?id=kwyF9vN6rwgC&pgis=1.

Doyal, L., & Pennell, I. 1979. *The Political Economy of Health.* Pluto Press.

Farley, J. 2003. *Bilharzia: A History of Imperial Tropical Medicine.* Cambridge University Press.

Farmer, P. E., Nizeye, B., Stulac, S., & Keshavjee, S. 2006. "Structural Violence and Clinical Medicine. *PLoS Medicine* 3 (10): e449. https://doi.org/10.1371/journal.pmed.0030449.

Farmer, P., Kim, J. Y., Kleinman, A., & Basilico, M. 2013. *Reimagining Global Health: An Introduction.* University of California Press.

Ferguson, J. 1994. *The Anti-Politics Machine: Development, Depoliticization, and Bureaucratic Power in Lesotho.* University of Minnesota Press.

Floridi, L. 2004. "Open Problems in the Philosophy of Information." *Metaphilosophy* 35 (4), 554–82. https://doi.org/10.1111/j.1467-9973.2004.00336.x.

Foucault, M. 1999. "Discourse and Truth: The Problematization of Parrhesia." Accessed May 16, 2016. https://foucault.info/parrhesia/.

Frickel, S., & Gross, N. 2005. "A General Theory of Scientific/Intellectual Movements." *American Sociological Review* 70 (2), 204–32. https://doi.org/10.1177/000312240507000202.

Fried, L. P., Bentley, M. E., Buekens, P., Burke, D. S., Frenk, J. J., Klag, M. J., & Spencer, H. C. 2010. "Global Health Is Public Health." *The Lancet (London)* 375 (9714): 535–7. https://doi.org/10.1016/S0140-6736(10)60203-6.

Gale, T. 2001. "Critical Policy Sociology: Historiography, Archaeology and Genealogy as Methods of Policy Analysis." *Journal of Education Policy* 16 (5), 379–93. https://doi.org/10.1080/02680930110071002.

Godin, B. 2006. "The Linear Model of Innovation: The Historical Construction of an Analytical Framework." *Science, Technology & Human Values*, 31 (6), 639–67. http://doi.org/10.1177/0162243906291865.

Godin, B., & Lane, J. P. 2013. "Pushes and Pulls: Hi(S)tory of the Demand Pull Model of Innovation." *Science, Technology & Human Values* 38 (5): 621–54. https://doi.org/10.1177/0162243912473163.

Goffman, E. 1974. *Frame Analysis: An Essay on the Organization of Experience.* Harper & Row.

Goldstein, J. 1999. "Emergence as a Construct: History and Issues." *Emergence* 1 (1): 49–72. https://doi.org/10.1207/s15327000em0101_4.

Grandin, K., Wormbs, N., & Widmalm, S. 2004. *The Science-Industry Nexus: History, Policy, Implications.* Science History Publications.

Gross, M. 2007. "The Unknown in Process: Dynamic Connections of Ignorance, Non-Knowledge and Related Concepts." *Current Sociology* 55 (5): 742–59. https://doi.org/10.1177/0011392107079928.

Guldi, J., & Armitage, D. 2014. *The History Manifesto.* https://books.google.ch/books/about/The_History_Manifesto.html?id=TjjooQEACAAJ&pgis=1.

Gusfield, J. 1976. "The Literary Rhetoric of Science: Comedy and Pathos in Drinking Driver Research." *American Sociological Review* 41 (1): 16. https://doi.org/10.2307/2094370.

Guston, D. H. 2010. "The Anticipatory Governance of Emerging Technologies." *Journal of the Korean Vacuum Society* 19 (6): 432–41. https://doi.org/10.5757/JKVS.2010.19.6.432.

Hackett, E. J., Amsterdamska, O., Lynch, M. E., & Wajcman, J. 2008. *The Handbook of Science and Technology Studies.* MIT Press.

Haddon, C., Devanny, J., Forsdick, C., & Thompson, A. 2015. "What Is the Value of History in Policymaking?" https://instituteforgovernment.org.uk/publications/what-value-history-policymaking.

Harman, S. 2012. *Global Health Governance.* Routledge. https://books.google.com/books?id=zuvGBQAAQBAJ&pgis=1.

Harman, S. 2014. "Ebola and the Politics of a Global Health Crisis." *E-International Relations.* https://e-ir.info/2014/10/20/ebola-and-the-politics-of-a-global-health-crisis/.

Hess, D. n.d. "Mobilized Publics, Science, and Technology." https://davidjhess.org/movements-and-publics.html.

Hekman, S. J. 1983. *Weber, the Ideal Type, and Contemporary Social Theory.* University of Notre Dame Press.

Hewlett, B. S., & Cline, B. L. 1997. "Anthropological Contributions to a Community-Based Schistosomiasis Control Project in Northern Cameroun. *Tropical Medicine & International Health: TM & IH* 2 (11), A25–36. https://ncbi.nlm.nih.gov/pubmed/9391520.

Hilgartner, S., & Bosk, C. L. 1988. "The Rise and Fall of Social Problems: A Public Arenas Model." *American Journal of Sociology* 94 (1), 53–78. https://doi.org/10.1086/228951.

Holland, Walter W., Olsen, J., & Florey, C. du V. 2007. *The Development of Modern Epidemiology: Personal Reports from Those Who Were There.* Oxford University Press.

IHME. n.d. "About." http://healthdata.org

Ikeda, S. 2002. *Dynamics of the Mixed Economy: Toward a Theory of Interventionism.* Routledge.

Illich, I. 1975. "The Medicalization of Life." *Journal of Medical Ethics* 1 (2): 73–7. https://doi.org/10.1136/jme.1.2.73.

Institute for Health Metrics and Evaluation. 2010. Projects.

Joly, P. B. 2010. "On the Economics of Technoscientific Promises, 203–222." https://researchgate.net/publication/277341791_On_the_economics_of_technoscientific_promises.

Kelly, A. H., & Beisel, U. 2011. "Neglected Malarias: The Frontlines and Back Alleys of Global Health." *BioSocieties* 6(S1): 71–87. https://doi.org/10.1057/biosoc.2010.42.

Kenny, K. E. 2015. "The Biopolitics of Global Health: Life and Death in Neoliberal Time." *Journal of Sociology* 51 (1): 9–27. https://doi.org/10.1177/1440783314562313.

Krumeich, A., Weijts, W., Reddy, P., & Meijer-Weitz, A. 2001. "The Benefits of Anthropological Approaches for Health Promotion Research and Practice." *Health Education Research* 16 (2): 121–30. https://doi.org/10.1093/her/16.2.121.

Latour, B. 2005. *Reassembling the Social: An Introduction to Actor-Network-Theory: An Introduction to Actor-Network-Theory.* Oxford University Press. https://books.google.co.uk/books/about/Reassembling_the_Social_An_Introduction.html?id=DlgNiBaYo-YC&pgis=1.

Lau, R. R., & Schlesinger, M. 2005. Policy "Frames, Metaphorical Reasoning, and Support for Public Policies." *Political Psychology* 26 (1): 77–114. https://doi.org/10.1111/j.1467-9221.2005.00410.x.

Lemaine, G., Macleod, R., Mulkay, M., Weingart, P., & Gruyter, W. de. 1976. *Perspectives on the Emergence of Scientific Disciplines.* Walter de Gruyter. https://books.google.co.uk/books/about/Perspectives_on_the_Emergence_of_Scienti.html?id=PfotstpTldoC&pgis=1.

Lindlof, T. R., & Taylor, B. C. 2011. *Qualitative Communication Research Methods.* Sage.

Majone, G. 1989. *Evidence, Argument, and Persuasion in the Policy Process.* Yale University Press.

Marmot, M. 2007. "Achieving Health Equity: From Root Causes to Fair Outcomes. *The Lancet* 370 (9593): 1153–63. https://doi.org/10.1016/S0140-6736(07)61385-3.

Marston, G., & Watts, R. 2003. "Tampering with the Evidence: A Critical Appraisal of Evidence-Based Policy-Making." *The Drawing Board: An Australian Review of Public Affairs* 3 (3): 143–63. https://researchbank.rmit.edu.au/view/rmit:7593.

Martin, S., & Scott, J. T. 2000. "The Nature of Innovation Market Failure and the Design of Public Support for Private Innovation." *Research Policy* 29 (4–5): 437–47.

McCloskey, D. N. 1998. *The Rhetoric of Economics.* University of Wisconsin Press.

McInnes, C., Kamradt-Scott, A., Lee, K., Reubi, D., Roemer-Mahler, A., Rushton, S., … Woodling, M. 2012. "Framing Global Health: The Governance Challenge." *Global Public Health* 7 (sup2): S83–S94. https://doi.org/10.1080/17441692.2012.733949.

Montresor, A., Gabrielli, A. F., Engels, D., Daumerie, D., & Savioli, L. 2013. "Has the NTD Community Neglected Evidence-Based Policy? PLOS NTDs 2013 Expert Commentary of the Viewpoint by Nagpal S, Sinclair D, Garner P." *PLoS Neglected Tropical Diseases* 7 (7): e2299. https://doi.org/10.1371/journal.pntd.0002299.

Moran, M., Guzman, J., Henderson, K., Liyanage, R., Wu, L., Chin, E., ... Kwong, D. 2012. *G-FINDER 2012: Neglected Disease Research & Development: A Five Year Review*. Policy Cures.

Morel, C. M. 2003. "Neglected Diseases: Under-Funded Research and Inadequate Health Interventions. Can We Change This Reality?" *EMBO Reports*, *4 Spec No*(6S) S35–8. https://doi.org/10.1038/sj.embor.embor851.

Mueller-Langer, F. 2013. "Neglected Infectious Diseases: Are Push and Pull Incentive Mechanisms Suitable for Promoting Drug Development Research?" *Health Economics, Policy, and Law* 8 (2), 185–208. https://doi.org/10.1017/S1744133112000321.

Muniesa, F., & Linhardt, D. 2009. *At Stake with Implementation: Trials of Explicitness in the Description of the State* (No. 015). Sociologie de L'Innovation Mines Paristech/CNRS UM.

Ng, N., & Ruger, J. 2011. "Global Health Governance at a Crossroads." *Global Health Governance*. http://search.ebscohost.com/login.aspx?direct=true&profile=ehost&scope=site&authtype=crawler&jrnl=19392389&AN=64305235&h=lg908ao62gGaJg2IGECbBbkw9xXdFYjJVTXjg6L04ZGEJcjf%2Bk%2BTngy266Y5ZYSPpL2GOcyKCz3JKGlKuxvk8Q%3D%3D&crl=c.

Oxford Dictionaries. n.d. "Problem – Definition of Problem in English." https://en.oxforddictionaries.com/definition/problem.

Parker, M., & Allen, T. 2011. "Does Mass Drug Administration for the Integrated Treatment of Neglected Tropical Diseases Really Work? Assessing Evidence for the Control of Schistosomiasis and Soil-Transmitted Helminths in Uganda." *Health Research Policy and Systems/BioMed Central* 9 (1): 3. https://doi.org/10.1186/1478-4505-9-3.

Parker, M., & Allen, T. 2013. "De-Politicizing Parasites: Reflections on Attempts to Control the Control of Neglected Tropical Diseases." http://dx.doi.org/10.1080/01459740.2013.831414.

Parker, M., Polman, K., & Allen, T. 2016. "Neglected Tropical Diseases in Biosocial Perspective." *Journal of Biosocial Science* 48(S1): S1–S15. https://doi.org/10.1017/S0021932016000274.

Pillemer, K., & Finkelhor, D. 1988. "The Prevalence of Elder Abuse: A Random Sample Survey." *The Gerontologist* 28 (1): 51–7. https://doi.org/10.1093/geront/28.1.51.

Policy Cures Research. 2020. "G-FINDER 2020 report. Neglected Tropical Disease Research and Development: Where to Now?" 2020. Available: https://policycuresresearch.org/analysis.

Popper, Karl R. 1957. *The Poverty of Historicism*. Routledge.

Proctor, R., & Schiebinger, L. L. 2008. *Agnotology: The Making and Unmaking of Ignorance*. Stanford University Press.

Ramalingam, B. 2014. "Navigating 'Wicked' Problems in Development." *ODI*.

Rappert, B., & Balmer, B. 2016. *Absence in Science, Security and Policy: From Research Agendas to Global Strategy*. Springer. https://books.google.com/books?id=S4-kCgAAQBAJ&pgis=1.

Reisz, M. 2013. "Unwanted Side-Effects." *The Times Higher Education*. May 30, 2013.

Rennie, R. 1998. "History and Policy-Making." *International Social Science Journal* 50 (156): 289–301. https://doi.org/10.1111/1468-2451.00131.

Restivo, S. 1988. "Modern Science as a Social Problem." *Social Problems* 35 (3). https://jstor.org/stable/800619?seq=1#page_scan_tab_contents.

Reynolds, A. 2008. "What Is Historicism?" http://dx.doi.org/10.1080/02698599 908573626.

Riecken, H. 1969. "Social Science and Contemporary Social Problems." http://items. ssrc.org/social-science-and-contemporary-social-problems/.

Rittel, H. W. J., & Webber, M. M. 1973. "Dilemmas in a General Theory of Planning." *Policy Sciences* 4 (2): 155–69. https://doi.org/10.1007/BF01405730.

Robbins, P. 2012. *Political Ecology: A Critical Introduction.* Wiley-Blackwell.

Rochefort, D. A., & Cobb, R. W. 1993. "Problem Definition, Agenda Access, and Policy Choice." *Policy Studies Journal* 21 (1): 56–71. https://doi.org/10.1111/j.1541-0072.1993.tb01453.x.

Rostow, W. W. 1971. *Politics and the Stages of Growth.* Cambridge Books.

Ruger, J. P. 2005. "The Changing Role of the World Bank in Global Health." *American Journal of Public Health* 95 (1): 60–70. https://doi.org/10.2105/AJPH.2004.042002.

Sanderson, I. 2002. "Evaluation, Policy Learning and Evidence-Based Policy Making." *Public Administration* 80 (1): 1–22. https://doi.org/10.1111/1467-9299.00292.

Schroeder, R. 2007. *Rethinking Science, Technology, and Social Change.* Stanford University Press.

Scoones, I. 2014. "The Politics of Trypanosomiasis Control in Africa." https:// opendocs.ids.ac.uk/opendocs/handle/20.500.12413/6700.

Sell, S. K., & Prakash, A. 2004. "Using Ideas Strategically: The Contest Between Business and NGO Networks in Intellectual Property Rights." *International Studies Quarterly* 48 (1): 143–75. https://doi.org/10.1111/j.0020-8833.2004.00295.x.

Simmons, B. A., Dobbin, F., & Garrett, G. 2007. "The Global Diffusion of Public Policies: Social Construction, Coercion, Competition or Learning?" Retrieved from http://papers.ssrn.com/abstract=1517972.

Steensland, B. 2008. "Why Do Policy Frames Change? Actor-Idea Coevolution in Debates over Welfare Reform." *Social Forces* 86 (3): 1027–54. https://doi.org/ 10.1353/sof.0.0027.

Stengers, I. 2015. *In Catastrophic Times.* Open Humanities Press/Meson Press.

Stilgoe, J. 2016. "Book Review: Nobody Knows Anything." *Issues in Science and Technology* 32 (4): 220. http://issues.org/32-4/book-review-nobody-knows-anything/.

Strydom, P. 1999. "The Challenge of Responsibility for Sociology." *Current Sociology* 47 (3): 65–82. https://doi.org/10.1177/0011392199047003006.

Thaler, R. H., & Sunstein, C. R. 2008. *Nudge: Improving Decisions about Health, Wealth, and Happiness.* Yale University Press.

Trouiller, P., Olliaro, P., Torreele, E., Orbinski, J., Laing, R., & Ford, N. 2002. "Drug Development for Neglected Diseases: A Deficient Market and a Public-Health Policy Failure. *The Lancet* 359 (9324): 2188–94. https://doi.org/10.1016/ S0140-6736(02)09096-7.

Tullock, G., Brady, G., & Seldon, A. 2002. *Government Failure: A Primer in Public Choice; Government's Greatest Achievements: From Civil Rights to Homeland Security.* Cato Institute. https://doi.org/978-1-935308-00-3.

Turnbull, N. 2008. "Harold Lasswell's 'Problem orientation' for the Policy Sciences." *Critical Policy Studies* 2 (1): 72–91. https://doi.org/10.1080/19460171.2008.9518532

Webster, A. 1991. *Science, Technology and Society: New Directions.* Palgrave Macmillan.

WHO. 2006. "Neglected Tropical Diseases: Hidden Successes, Emerging Opportunities." Accessed August 6, 2015. http://apps.who.int/iris/bitstream/10665/69367/1/WHO_CDS_NTD_2006.2_eng.pdf.

WHO. 2013. "World Health Assembly Adopts Resolution on All 17 Neglected Tropical Diseases." *World Health Organisation.* https://who.int/neglected_diseases/WHA_66_seventh_day_resolution_adopted/en/.

Zahariadis, N. 2016. *Handbook of Public Policy Agenda Setting.* Edward Elgar Publishing.

Zhang, D., Unschuld, P. U., Li, T., Chen, H., Mao, Z., Anon, … Zhang, Z. 2008. "China's Barefoot Doctor: Past, Present, and Future." *The Lancet* 372 (9653): 1865–67. https://doi.org/10.1016/S0140-6736(08)61355-0.

Chapter 3

The politics of disease categories

A history of NTDs as a policy issue

Beginning in the 1970s, I will explore the history of neglected tropical diseases (NTDs) by primarily using a comparison of two early initiatives that spurred advocacy at the WHO and Rockefeller Foundation and were precursors for the NTD concept. I am interested in the context for how policy thinking changed over time and why the current conceptualisation of NTDs did not arise directly through the WHO. I will provide a background of the key events, actors, institutions, initiatives, the coining of the term, and the changing classificatory lists of diseases that constituted NTDs – which diseases have counted as NTDs and why. The ambivalence of categorisations of NTDs is due to finding coherent criteria for inclusion or exclusion that also has policy appeal. I discuss the reasoning behind the different lists and show how country or regional NTD characteristics challenge an all-encompassing view, concluding with a discussion about the strategies of policy influence that came to dominate. The targeting of intervention on five NTDs led to some of the diseases being described as 'tool-ready'. The dominant strategies to treat NTDs came from global campaigns including the Sustainable Development Goals (SDGs) and the emergence of new institutions, including the work of the Gates Foundation, focusing on drug donation and R&D to tackle NTDs.

Before tackling these issues, it is crucial to look at the NTD term for how 'neglect' is understood. The question this chapter and following chapters will be preoccupied with is why and by whom neglect is originated and perpetuated, and the attempts made to redress neglect. The broad categories of neglect have been an early point addressed in the academic literature (see Holt, Gillam, & Ngondi, 2012; Liese & Schubert, 2009; Morel et al., 2005). These categories are centred on science (universities, research institutes), the market (pharmaceutical companies), and public health (donors, international organisations, philanthropy).

The group that has been consistently active in its commitment to and also in encouraging a renewed interest in NTDs is the donor community. Big pharma, on the other hand, has faced pressure to address issues of global health, and this influenced their increased involvement, through donation programmes. The result has been that more pharma companies donated drugs as part of their corporate social responsibility obligations. However, the pharmaceutical industry did not form a concerted advocacy campaign or an expansion of attention towards NTDs.

Early initiatives: 'bringing science into tropical disease research'

The donor community in the 1970s marked out the territory for NTD policy through initiatives by the major global health actors – the Rockefeller Foundation and the WHO. The Rockefeller Foundation was established in 1909 as the Rockefeller Sanitary Commission – a philanthropic organisation funded with an endowment of $3.4bn from JD Rockefeller Sr.'s incredibly profitable Standard Oil Company, founded in the 1870s (Farley, 2004). Rockefeller had as his principal aid in philanthropy a former businessman and Baptist minister, Frederick Gates, who decided upon a medical focus. Gates had felt medicine to be a neglected area that deserved more attention:

> … 'I had begun to realize how woefully neglected had been the scientific study of medicine in the United States'. What was needed, he concluded, was a research institute given to 'uninterrupted study and investigation, on ample salary, entirely independent of practice' ….
>
> (ibid., p. 3)

It was an example of scientization[1] of medicine with a desire to scale up funding in an independent and exploratory laboratory setting, away from patients, hospitals, and the 'practice' of health. Gates also indicated a need to concentrate on a neglected topic.

Scientific research as a philanthropic 'cause' may sound unusual, but many of the most well-established and well-funded philanthropic organisations have this as their mission.[2] In an era before big science projects of national importance, during and after World War II, and when major government funding organisations were in their infancy, philanthropy also played a crucial role for research.[3] Global health efforts were more of a rarity before the post-war era, and as a result coordination on a worldwide scale would come to the health realm relatively late. The WHO was established as a specialised agency of UN concerned with international public health in 1948, stemming from the earlier League of Nations Health Organization (LNHO), which had been modelled on the Rockefeller Foundation (Borowy, 2009). Arguably, the WHO's largest and most successful role has been in the global campaign for the eradication of smallpox, yet the initial priorities were wide-ranging: "malaria, tuberculosis, venereal diseases, maternal and child health, sanitary engineering, and nutrition" (McCarthy, 2002, p. 1111).

It would be much later in the histories of the Rockefeller Foundation and the WHO – during the 1970s to 1990s – that the preparatory groundwork was set for the creation of NTDs. The first initiative, established by the WHO, was the Special Programme for Research and Training in Tropical Diseases (TDR) (1974–present). The Rockefeller Foundation established the second major NTD initiative, the 'Great Neglected Diseases of Mankind' – GND (1978–1988). Separate analyses have been conducted on these initiatives (Farley, 2004; Keating, 2014; Remme et al., 2002; Zhou, Wayling, & Bergquist, 2010), however, their purposes were similar.

Both were premised on bringing science into research for tropical diseases through 'capacity-building' meaning building the scientific expertise and research capabilities of those working on NTDs, particularly in low- and middle-income countries, by providing the support and network of high-income countries. The driving goal of the TDR was to develop new drugs (and other innovations) for neglected infectious diseases in low- and middle-income countries and have their scientists advance their research skills.[4] In line with a capacity-building approach, the endemic country took centre stage – although this did still assume a transfer of knowledge and resources from high-income to low- and middle-income countries. For the GND, the goal was also to develop drugs for neglected diseases, but with a greater emphasis on basic research and the introduction of new scientific techniques.

The diseases that the initiatives included both hold similarities with the current NTD grouping. The TDR included seven diseases that would later be included in the first WHO list of 13 NTDs (with the exception of malaria). At the time, the first director of the TDR, Adetokunbo Lucas, noted: "These diseases were selected by the criteria of their public health importance, the lack of effective tools for their control, and the likelihood that research can yield the new tools which could bring significant advances in their control" (Fudenberg, 1983, p. 160). As of 2020, the TDR also includes malaria, Ebola, and TB, in addition to the WHO NTDs. The TDR does not make the distinction of malaria and TB being relatively less neglected as part of the Big Three and nor is Ebola out of scope as an emerging disease. As the focus is on capacity-building and scientific progress, there is still much to be achieved for these diseases. Rockefeller's GND – also included diseases not typically described as NTDs, such as diarrheal diseases and other typical diseases of poverty not especially tropical by nature (see Table 3.1 below for a comparison of the diseases covered by the TDR, in both 1978 and 2016, and the GND in 1978).

It would be much later that the WHO latched onto neglected as a descriptor for tropical diseases. The WHO made references to neglect but this tended to be as a rhetorical device, as described by the WHO in 1990: "Human commitment and resources are required of the world, if tropical diseases are

Table 3.1 Comparing TDR diseases to GND diseases

	TDR 1978	TDR 2016	GND 1978
Chagas disease	x	x	
Dengue		x	
Diarrheal diseases			x
Ebola		x	
Filariasis (inc. lymphatic filariasis and onchocerciasis)	x	x	
HAT	x	x	
Helminthiasis (inc. hookworm)		x	x
Leishmaniasis	x	x	
Leprosy	x	x	
Malaria	x	x	x
Schistosomiasis	x	x	x
TB		x	

(US Congress Office of Technology Assessment, 1985; Lucas, 2013)

not to become the great *neglected* diseases of mankind" (WHO TDR-CTD; emphasis added). While the TDR may initially appear to be the natural home for the creation of NTDs, this proved not to be the case. According to one of the advocate scientists:

> ... TDR I think dropped the ball ... They lost the disease focus ... the point is that TDR never invented or had anything to do with the concept of NTDs ... they were involved in some excellent work on oncho[5] ... they did fundamental early work ... TDR are basically an organisation that take donor money and redistribute it, the work is done by scientists who apply for grants.
> (interview with author, scientist advocate, 2016)

In losing the 'disease focus', what is being implied is that the TDR became more concerned with the distribution of donor money and encouraging capacity-building of scientists. This account is one explicit statement about the lack of WHO involvement in originating the concept of NTDs but is reflected from other informants. The point they made was that the WHO is not well placed for advocacy and conceptual input into disease issues. As Nick Kourgialis from Helen Keller International (an organisation concerned with causes and consequences of blindness and malnutrition) explained: "So they're a critical partner but I'm not sure that they've been as directly involved with or important in the advocacy that occurs on the country level, in the US, in the UK and others" (interview with author, Kourgialis, 2016). Their role was more centred on setting global standards and criteria (e.g. elimination) for reporting and guidance on clinical protocols to highlight the importance of issues and providing a forum for discussions and assessing progress. Therefore, it is clear that while providing early leadership on policy and scientific research, the TDR were not involved in the conceptual construct of NTDs. Some institutional groundwork was laid as tropical diseases were embedded early on in the WHO machinery.

As Keusch writes (in Parker & Sommer, 2010), the TDR was a somewhat unique entity within the WHO, as a partnership with the United Nations Development Programme (UNDP) and the World Bank. The TDR had more independence in being supported by external funds, so that it could determine how to put resources to use without interference from WHO leadership and was determined to keep a degree of independence (ibid.).[6] This reliance on external funds and partners, and encouragement of drug donation, also may have opened the door for private sector and philanthropic actors to become involved later.[7]

Institutionally, the Rockefeller Foundation did not have to reach the type of consensus that the WHO needed as a multi-constituency representative body. Still, scientific research capacity-building was a main pursuit of both programmes. The GND at the time of its operation was heavily interested in attracting the 'crème de la crème' of scientific talent, and was more agnostic about whether that was in high-income or low- and middle-income countries. In a profile on the WHO website, Lucas (2013 [1978], p. 220) stated how he was hopeful at inception that the TDR "... will produce results which would otherwise not have been attained through the traditional isolated and disjointed approach to such problems" (Fleck, 2015, pp. 292–3). The TDR wanted to produce scientific results specifically via low- and middle-income countries by building their talent base (see Fleck, 2015; Lucas, 2013). Also, expectations for new biotechnological advances to solve old problems were high, as Lucas described:

> ... the vigorous application of recent advances in modern biology would yield a better understanding of parasites and parasitism ... an interdisciplinary approach using the modern tools of research in immunology, histochemistry, biochemistry, molecular biology, genetics ... by focusing attention of scientists on the needs and opportunities for research in this area, more rapid progress can be made.
>
> (2013 [1978], p. 220)

The scientific focus, especially the application of new scientific specialties, would become less pronounced and was certainly a perceived need in the 1970s in both GND and TDR.

At the WHO, the TDR focus in later years moved onto how research could support and improve health outcomes, as opposed to an exploratory introduction of biotechnology. The director since 2012, John Reeder, explained in an interview with the UN-associated news website *Genève Internationale*[8] that, "… really, it's about putting research into the service of improving people's health" (Genève Internationale, 2014). This outlook is a concern for implementation, and operational research, to consider country capacity, delivery, and uptake. Reeder argued that it differed from when they started, as there were "many new medicines and diagnostic tools, but they aren't always getting to the people who need them … Our strategic shift has been downstream towards the diseases in country" (ibid.).

Bernadette Ramirez – a scientist working in Reeder's unit – described how, as part of financial prioritisation at the WHO, TDR underwent a "refocus of strategy in light of limited resources and reprioritization exercise" (interview with author, 2013). The focus would remain on capacity-building, "… looking at current gaps to add value for the needs of the community" (ibid.). In terms of involvement in cutting-edge research, she explained the view that there already was enough: "… capacity on the ground as far as [drug] discovery" (ibid.). TDR could facilitate 'R&D mapping' and research networks had been set up and were embedded in disease endemic countries but they were "… no longer pursuing drug discovery as a major activity" (ibid.). The overall approach, in attracting the best scientific talent, would have the biggest legacy. The TDR and GND, and their institutional setting, show how the ground was set for the concept of NTDs to emerge. While the WHO was unable to be the originator of NTDs because its advocacy ability was limited, the GND would be the conceptual origin for NTDs. Next, I consider the ongoing role of the WHO and the Rockefeller Foundation, and what the GND and TDR say about the transition from tropical disease, missing from largely historical accounts (Hotez et al., 2012; Lammie et al., 2007), and look towards the new configuration of tropical diseases as NTDs.

The WHO has been criticised for not paying enough attention to diseases of the poor. While the TDR could also be seen as a return to the original goal of 'health for all' (Gillam, 2008) in not forgetting the poorest communities, for some this ambition did not go far enough.[9] This was certainly the view of Kenneth Warren, the director of the GND, that the WHO had not concentrated on "… those few diseases that caused the highest mortality among the world's poor" (Keating, 2014, S.25). Also, the limited advocacy role by the WHO is still acknowledged. Kari Stoever, at the 'Global Network for Neglected Tropical Diseases', one of the main advocacy NGOs established in 2006, spoke of the difficult position the WHO held:

> … because of the way they're set up to be a bureaucracy and to gain consensus and when you're an advocate you've got to drive to a goal and it's usually very short term … you're trying to push the needle faster than

the WHO would be able to convene or develop consensus among their members.

(interview with author, Stoever, 2016)

It has been the case that from inception in 1948 until the late 1990s, the WHO fared variably, described as moving:

> ... from a commanding position as the unquestioned leader of international health to a much-diminished role in the crowded and contested world of global health ... WHO was marked from its early days by political and diplomatic entanglements and budgetary constraints that, over five decades, compromised the organization and restricted its operating capacity. Indeed, those entanglements and constraints eventually pushed WHO in the 1990s to try to reinvent itself as a coordinator of global health in a world with many new and powerful players.
>
> (Brown & Cueto in Parker & Sommer, 2010, p. 18)

The Rockefeller Foundation then suffered from a change in topics of focus, which is why it has not had a continued influence with NTDs. Chen remarks on how "(F)oundations are strange creatures since they are not driven by the accountability of the ballot box, scrutiny of the media, or even restrictive regulations" (2014, p. 719). The topics of focus are often directed by the individual preferences of the foundation.

Before the launch of the GND, the Rockefeller Foundation had been concerned with agricultural science[10] and population growth.[11] The programmes in health sciences, which had been the flagship programmes at the foundation's creation, had already diminished by the 1970s. Today population growth is not viewed as such a major concern; but in the 1960s and 1970s, population growth was seen as a great threat to high-income countries, as shown by such dystopian sci-fi films as 'Soylent Green' released in 1973, imagining some of the horrors of too many people scrambling for limited resources (Haberman, 2015). This anxiety about the population growing faster than available resources also predated the green revolution of high-yielding, disease-resistant crops, and the rapid economic growth of low- and middle-income countries such as Brazil and India, which later saw declines in birth rate growth (ibid.).[12]

The Division of Health Sciences at the Rockefeller Foundation reflected these popular sentiments, prevalent in academic circles and the public imagination. However, the division would experience changes that would bring traditional health concerns back into the picture. Four key members of the division had retired, opening the door for a change of direction (Kreier, 2014). As Warren remarked, because of, "... the relative lack of constraints upon voluntary organizations, this could have been in many different directions", but the leadership of the director, John H. Knowles, had set this focus on health (ibid., p. 336). The topic of focus was to be: "… the major diseases of the forgotten three-quarters of the world's people in developing countries" and, in a sense, a return to the foundation's roots, as it had begun with a major global hookworm campaign (ibid.).

Both the TDR and GND had returned, through these initiatives to the founding ideals of their institutions, but were also keen to leave behind 'colonial baggage', and mark a discontinuity with colonial health and the beginning of a new global health. It is ironic as Rockefeller had been accused of a new colonialism in pursuing US interests through the earlier hookworm campaigns (McGoey, 2015a) but the GND has not been accused of a similar agenda. As Chapter 4 discusses further, a previous colonial shaping of tropical diseases meant that in the post-colonial era a new approach would be sought. The TDR and GND signalled a way to go about to addressing tropical diseases that differed from the colonial campaigns that existed until most countries achieved independence by the 1970s. Although the colonial history is a lingering point (even in the names of the initiatives), the TDR kept 'tropical diseases' in its name and mission statement. The TDR director in 2007, Robert Ridley, defended the decision years later in a profile on the WHO website:

Q: The concept of 'tropical diseases' originates from the medicine practiced by 19th century colonial powers to protect themselves in the tropics. Have you considered changing your name?

A: There has been some discussion about the name. Our new strategy refers more to 'infectious diseases of poverty', but if you look at the terms 'tropical disease and tropical medicine', they still cover a field that is generally recognized today. You still have associations and institutes with the name and – at the WHO – a department of neglected tropical diseases. The name has other connotations which we should be aware of, but given the recognition of the name and loyalty to TDR, particularly in developing countries, we decided to keep it.

(Bulletin of the World Health Organization, 2007)

The GND, on the other hand, chose to rename what was largely a group of tropical diseases, to emphasise the common humanity implicated in 'diseases of mankind'[13] and the scale and problem of 'the great neglected'.[14] Maybe it had been the historian in Warren (who had studied history and literature before switching to medicine), as director of the GND, who proposed the title. The word 'great' had been used in tropical medicine to elevate the importance, – scientifically and to society of tackling these diseases, – just as 'neglected' would similarly be used in an instrumental way, this time to highlight moral obligation and need. The wording 'mankind' was a part of what the foundation was about, "to promote the well being of mankind throughout the world" (Birn et al., 2013, p. 1618).

In the next section, I look towards the reasons why new activities and organisational structures have been required to further the NTD cause, a symptom also of the change in global health. The WHO has been both an influential entity and a bureaucratic institution that many did not view as an advocacy organisation. After the launch of the TDR, the WHO endured a 'declining role', confounded by the relative ascendance of the World Bank, which was able to intervene more actively in world health affairs through 'structural adjustment policies' that tied health to the economy and financial support (Kenny, 2015). The organisation has also had to contend with new entrants into global health, particularly from the early 2000s onward.

Similarly, the Rockefeller Foundation, after some initial success with the GND programme, would find it difficult to maintain relevance following the proliferation of global governance institutions. From the WHO and other UN agencies to the World Bank, widening the health focus in their activities, both institutions would face increased competition. After the turn of this century, the Rockefeller Foundation would be overtaken by the Gates Foundation as the foremost philanthropic donor in public health. Therefore, while both institutions contributed towards the NTD policy cause, it would take a very different set of actors to take tropical diseases forward in a new global health landscape.

Timeline of key events

The stage was then set for a number of milestones in the creation of NTDs as a policy and disease category, after the 'Millennium Development Goals' (MDGs) in 2000 – from the first NTD paper in 2004 to the Berlin meeting in 2005, quickly followed by the creation of the WHO department for NTDs and the first WHO report on NTDs. This collection of milestones then reached a pinnacle with a landmark event in 2012, 'The London Declaration', and the formal instillation of NTDs on policy agendas through the 2015 Sustainable Development Goals (SDGs). See below a timeline of these key events (Figure 3.1).

From the Berlin meeting to the London Declaration

A 'historical meeting in Berlin' took place between 18 and 20 April 2005 (Savioli, Montresor, & Gabrielli, 2011, p. 486). WHO representatives Savioli, Montresor, and Gabrielli from the Department of Control of Neglected Tropical Diseases describe it as when the WHO "… formally rebranded this area of work, previously vaguely defined as 'other communicable diseases' or 'other tropical diseases', meaning other than malaria, tuberculosis, and HIV/AIDS, as neglected tropical diseases" (ibid.). Scientist advocate Alan

> ### 1970s - 1990s Pre-MDGs
>
> GND (1978 – 1988), TDR (1974 – present)

> ### 2000 MDGs
>
> Gavi, the Vaccine Alliance (2000), The Global Fund to fight AIDS,
> Tuberculosis and Malaria (2002)

> ### 2003 NTD branding and funding
>
> First Berlin Meeting (2003), First NTD paper (2004), WHO Department for NTDs
> (2005), The Global Network for NTDs (2006), PLOS Neglected Tropical Diseases
> (2007), G8 Meeting in Japan (2008), Presidential Initiative on NTDs and DFID
> Committment (2008), Bill & Melinda Gates Foundation funds Global Network
> (2009), First WHO report (2010)

2012 The London Declaration and WHO Roadmap

2015 SDGs

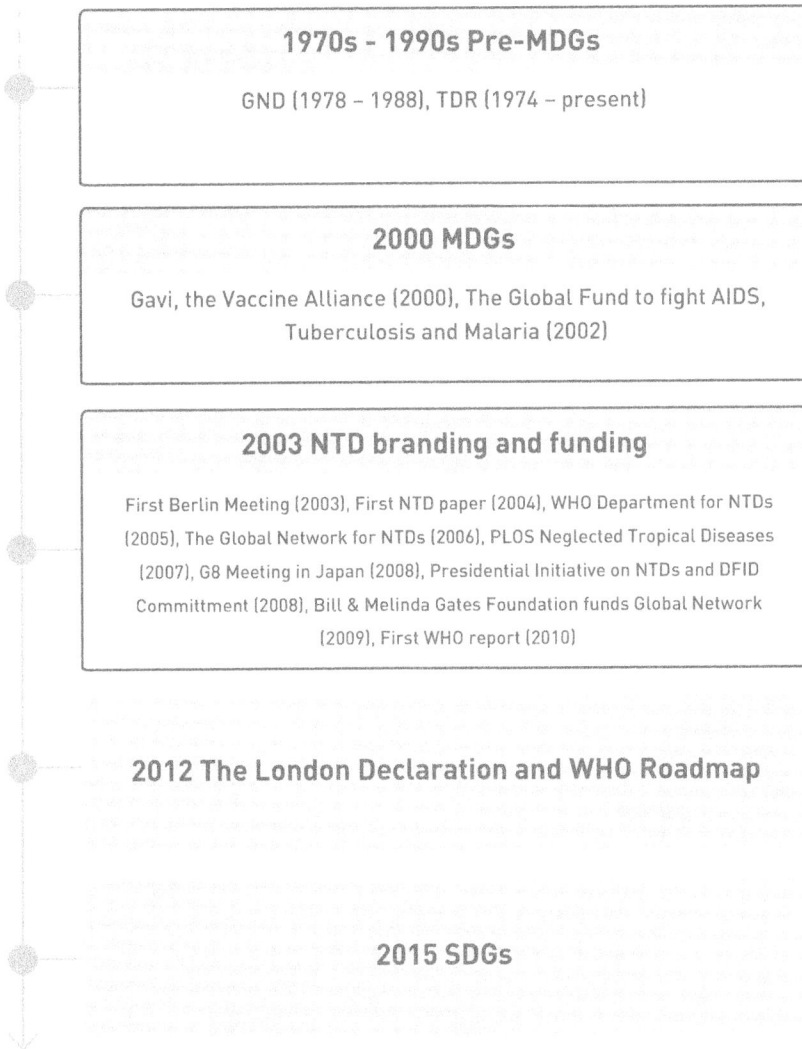

Figure 3.1 Timeline of main events in creation of NTDs from 1970 to 2015.

Fenwick also argued that it was at the meeting that much of the groundwork and discussions for coining NTDs happened:

> … it was a mixture of people who were interested in the various diseases and a selection of African Ministers of Health and whatnot, and we sat down and we talked, and we said what are we going to do? … And so the big question came up, can we integrate what we're doing and who the hell

can pronounce all these names? I'm the only one who can pronounce all these names and spell them. And so we needed a collective phrase and we discussed a number of different phrases and neglected topical diseases was the one that was selected, NTDs.

(interview with author, Fenwick, 2015)[15]

This international workshop was intended to be a 'Strategic and technical meeting on intensified control of neglected tropical diseases' (WHO, 2005). It was co-hosted by the WHO, the German Ministry for Economic Cooperation and Development, the German Ministry of Health, Deutsche Gesellshaft für Technische Zusammenarbeit (GTZ), Kredinstalt für Wiederaufbau (KFW), and the TDR.[16] Present were experts from public health, economics, and human rights, which explain the focus on these areas in the proceeding report (ibid.). Molyneux describes how:

... Dr Anarfi Asamoa-Baah, now the Deputy Director General [at the WHO], was at that meeting and decided he would create the department ... He said I'm going to do it tomorrow ... so that's when it happened that the Department at the WHO was created.

(interview with author, scientist advocate, 2016)

The meeting coordinated efforts towards a new strategic approach. Savioli et al. called this a paradigm change within the WHO:

In 2003, under the leadership of Dr. J. W. Lee, just appointed Director General, the World Health Organization (WHO) started a process of paradigm shift in the control and elimination of neglected tropical diseases (NTDs). The shift consisted of the adoption of a new vision that abandoned a purely academic approach to adopt one more responsive to the needs of affected individuals and communities. As a consequence, it entailed a strategic rethinking and a move away from a 'theoretical,' structural classification based on disease biology toward a 'practical' one based on the available tools employed to control such diseases.

(Relman & Choffnes, 2011, p. 481)

The shift was based on the new drug strategy of preventative chemotherapy through Mass Drug Administration (or MDA). As described by Savioli, attention was directed towards policy design and outcomes rather than a technical approach considering the diseases separately. The door was also opened to consider a societal understanding and apply a social science lens with economics and human rights, and also public health, as both a "science and art of preventing disease, prolonging life and promoting health" (Acheson, 1988).[17]

The first paper

The Berlin meeting was an occasion for the term NTDs to come into being as the best descriptor of a group of tropical diseases that multiple partners were working on, with agreement among many of the central stakeholders. However, the term still needed further conceptualisation and promotion. The first paper most explicitly referring to NTDs, and which would prove influential in considering the policy intervention of NTDs, was "'Rapid-impact interventions': how a policy of integrated control for Africa's neglected tropical diseases could benefit the poor" (Molyneux, Hotez, & Fenwick, 2005).[18] The authors were David Molyneux, Peter Hotez, and Alan Fenwick, for *PLOS Medicine* in 2005. They questioned the lack of attention for the successes of NTD interventions from policymakers, donors, and public health officials. The vertical programmes were working well but could be combined for 'integrated control' and 'rapid impact'. Synergies could be produced by combining delivery of four drugs in a 'rapid impact package' aimed at five[19] NTDs (schistosomiasis, trachoma, lymphatic filariasis, onchocerciasis, and soil-transmitted helminths).

These diseases could be treated through the same drugs or delivered through a similar treatment (MDA), especially as at-risk populations often suffered from more than one disease in any case, with cost-effectiveness results.[20] The NGO 'Global Network for Neglected Tropical Diseases' calls this 'The Solution' on their webpage:

> We have the tools available to defeat the most common neglected trop-
> ical diseases (NTDs), and we can do it in our lifetime. Unlike many other
> global health problems we face today, the solution is relatively simple. For
> just 50 cents, we can provide a person with treatment against the most
> common NTDs for an entire year.
>
> (Global Network, n.d.)

Molyneux stated that the most important paper where he put down his thoughts about neglect and the successes achieved was already published in 2004, in *The Lancet*. The paper was titled: "'Neglected' diseases but unrecognized successes – challenges and opportunities for infectious disease control".[21] His primary motivational argument was that there already existed successful interventions that were not being sufficiently implemented. Therefore, it was the interventions and their success that were being neglected, not the diseases per se. The contrast Molyneux wanted to make was the 'inherent difficulty' in controlling the Big Three as opposed to the relative ease of controlling 'chronic biologically stable disabling infections' (Molyneux, 2004, p. 382). For him, the MDGs served as a rhetorical device to demonstrate NTDs had been sidelined in funding streams and priority setting. Therefore, according to Molyneux, the MDG argument was applied post hoc and was not itself a spur for activity. He was surprised by the reaction to his 2004 paper and the paper with Hotez and Fenwick in how the term NTD caught on:

> ... None of this was done deliberately ... when I wrote that paper in 2004 and then it just then took off, it resonated because we were struggling ... we couldn't persuade a donor, be it a bilateral donor ... to actually buy-in to the concept of a single disease, we had to find another thing and I was frustrated ... from 2004 to significant contributions from a whole range of parties ... effective partnerships across the patch, I certainly would have dreamt of almost 12 years afterwards from first paper, completely unthinkable.
>
> (second interview with author, Molyneux, 2016)

The single diseases stood up poorly to the big three and so the MDGs would later form a useful marker from which to provide evidence that NTDs were neglected. Perhaps more concerning to Molyneux was the excessive interest in emerging and re-emerging infectious diseases perceived as a threat (Ebola, West Nile virus, Nipah virus, and SARS), but a low significance in global public health terms (burden of disease) demonstrated by DALYs attributed (ibid., p. 180). Overall, these academic contributions were policy engaged and orientated, and followed by many papers about NTDs, with the authors describing what their view of the state of affairs and what should be done. Further thought development and action came in the establishment of *PLOS Neglected Tropical Diseases* journal in 2007, the G8 Meeting in Japan in 2008 which set NTDs as a priority, the Presidential Initiative on NTDs and DFID Commitment also in 2008, and the first WHO report on NTDs in 2010.

The London Declaration and disease lists

A culmination of events occurred on 30 January 2012 at 'The London Declaration' when international politicians, pharmaceutical CEOs, and heads of global health organisations (including Bill Gates and the Director of the World Health Organization, Margaret Chan) descended on London. This gathering of leaders was marked by the presence of big pharma, led by Bill Gates through the philanthropic Bill & Melinda Gates Foundation. Gates was already completely changing the landscape of public health through his $39.6 billion endowment to the foundation[22] and priorities set in the areas of health, development, and education. By the account of Molyneux, Gates was central, but there were others who also made the London Declaration happen: "It was DIFID[23] and Gates ... supported by pharma partners particularly by Andrew Whitty from GSK[24] with Lorenzo Savioli driving the agenda from the WHO side" (first interview with author, Molyneux, 2016).

This was a meeting for setting goals and forming a collective vision to tackle NTDs, echoing the Millennium Development Goals (MDGs) 12 years before. The MDGs were eight targets set to be reached by 2015, addressing the needs of the world's poorest people and agreed by all countries at UN. The London Declaration was reminiscent of the MDGs, though directed specifically at NTDs. Many highlighted the omission by the MDGs and how donor attention and funding was directed towards the Big Three. As Molyneux describes, policymakers and politicians "… overfocus on unachievable objectives and targets around the Big Three diseases, which if the planet was viewed by aliens would be seen as the only diseases that existed on the planet" (2008, p. 509).

At the London Declaration, only 10 NTDs were addressed, as the signatories decided that it was these which could be controlled or eliminated by the end of the decade: the diseases ripe for 'immediate targeted assistance'. This scope was in line with the early papers about integrating successful vertical programmes and explains the pharma company involvement. What the London Declaration was really about was the continuation of existing drug donation and research programmes with some encouragement of further R&D, the goals summarised as follows:

- sustain, expand and extend programmes, drug supply, and access
- advance R&D, collaboration/coordination
- funding for implementation and technical support to evaluate and monitor the interventions

Through a public announcement of commitments to NTDs, the intention was to address shortfalls in drug donations and to coordinate action by 2020. NTDs were described as such:

> These diseases, many of which have afflicted humanity for millennia, affect more than 1.4 billion people. They sicken, disable, and disfigure, keeping people in cycles of poverty and costing developing economies billions of dollars every year. Until recently, NTDs saw little attention from all but a small handful of dedicated supporters. But as their impact grew clearer, more were urged into action.
>
> (Uniting to Combat NTDs, 2014, p. 4)

This is a typical description of NTDs as diseases of and causing poverty that have been around a long time (some for millennia), disabling and disfiguring more than killing, still affecting many with an impact on their economies. The final point acknowledges that NTDs have been a neglected problem, but the situation is improving. There are a number of diseases that can be included in this group, although it is striking there is no global consensus on what these diseases are, nor any standardised definition, with different organisations defining these diseases differently.

Other organisations' disease lists also tend to have lower, more manageable numbers than the 20 making up the WHO list, with the exception of the 38 for open-access journal *PLOS Neglected Tropical Diseases*, established in 2007 through a $1.1 million grant from the Gates Foundation and with Peter Hotez as the founding Editor-and-Chief (The Official PLOS Blog, n.d.). It has a science, policy and advocacy mission, with a focus on the poverty and chronic aspect of NTDs impacting on "… child health and development, pregnancy, and worker productivity, as well as their stigmatizing features" (PLOS Neglected Tropical Diseases, n.d.). As an academic endeavour the journal has more reason for a wide scope and is open to the inclusion of other diseases with appropriate rationale. In addition to the WHO 20 are many viral and bacterial diseases, including some that were originally listed by Patrick Manson (see Manson, 1898), discussed in greater detail in Chapter 4.

The variation in the number of diseases is representative of how NTDs are diversely described and is not a purely biomedical description but related to several social characteristics, such as poverty, stigma, and voicelessness. Teasing out ideas about why certain categories or characterisations are used and the different ways of dividing up diseases, provides insight into the criteria determining which diseases are included and why.

Different ways to cut a pie

The WHO commonly distinguished NTDs by pathogen – ranging from viral (dengue fever and rabies) and bacterial (leprosy and blinding trachoma) to the less well-known protozoa diseases, including Chagas (closely linked with Latin America), and African sleeping sickness (only affecting sub-Saharan Africa). Then there is a large group of helminths (worms, such as guinea worm, lymphatic filariasis, and schistosomiasis); see Figure 3.2 below.

Another distinction is coverage by geographic region, for which diseases are most prevalent and where. Table 3.2 divides NTDs by specificities and priorities of WHO region.[25] This list has not been updated since five NTDs were more recently added, but it is still true that Africa has the highest number of NTDs, followed by the Americas, which have two tiers of specificities and priorities and where Chagas is unique. South East Asia, which has many high-income countries in the region, has NTDs that are targeted for elimination. The European and Eastern Mediterranean regions, as to be expected, have lower levels of NTDs and the severity is lower, including 'other zoonic diseases' in the table as well as anthrax and brucellosis, not typically classed as NTDs. These country and regional NTD characteristics challenge an all-encompassing view of the diseases. NTDs as a category applied to the African region is appropriate as this is a region with many; but for other regions,

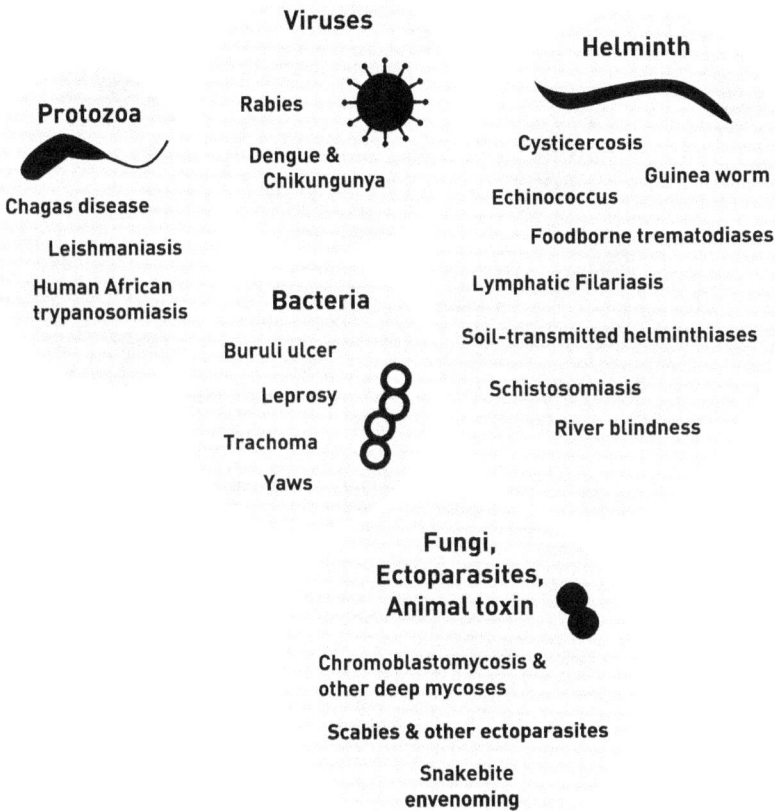

Viruses

Helminth

Protozoa

Rabies

Cysticercosis

Dengue &
Chikungunya

Guinea worm

Echinococcus

Chagas disease

Foodborne trematodiases

Leishmaniasis

Human African
trypanosomiasis

Lymphatic Filariasis

Bacteria

Soil-transmitted helminthiases

Buruli ulcer

Leprosy

Schistosomiasis

River blindness

Trachoma

Yaws

**Fungi,
Ectoparasites,
Animal toxin**

Chromoblastomycosis &
other deep mycoses

Scabies & other ectoparasites

Snakebite
envenoming

Figure 3.2 NTDs by pathogen.

(Adapted from Cotton, 2015)

the number of NTDs is limited, and so diseases have a regional character. However, it is the individual diseases themselves that make the NTD grouping the most unclear, contentious, and debatable – a point explored in the next section.

Listing diseases and the politics of categorisation

As Rosenberg describes, "… disease classifications serve to rationalize, mediate, and legitimate relationships between individuals and institutions in a bureaucratic society" (Rosenberg & Golden, 1992, pp. xxi). What is at stake in listing diseases and what are the consequences of the creation of categories

Table 3.2 NTDs by region

Specificities and priorities by WHO region	
Africa	Blinding trachoma
	Buruli ulcer
	Cysticercosis
	Dracunculiasis
	Echinococcosis
	Human African trypanosomiasis
	Leishmaniases
	Leprosy
	Lymphatic filariasis
	Onchocerciasis
	Rabies
	Schistosomiases
	Soil-transmitted helminthiasis
	Yaws
The Americas	***First tier***
	Blinding trachoma
	Chagas disease
	Leprosy
	Lymphatic filariasis
	Onchocerciasis
	Schistosomiasis
	Soil-transmitted helminthiasis
	Second tier
	Fungal and ectoparasitic skin diseases
	Leishmaniasis
	Parasitic zoonoses
The Eastern Mediterranean	Leishmaniases
	Schistosomiases
	Soil-transmitted helminthiasis
	Rabies
	Other zoonotic diseases
European	Anthrax
	Brucellosis
	Rabies
	Soil-transmitted helminthiasis
	Tularaemia
South-East Asia	***Diseases targeted for elimination***
	Anthroponotic leishmaniasis (kala-azar)
	Leprosy
	Lymphatic filariasis
	Yaws
The Western Pacific	Dengue
	Lymphatic filariasis
	Schistosomiasis
	Soil-transmitted

(WHO, 2007, p. 3)

to include or exclude? Five diseases targeted by United States Agency for International Development (USAID with the project ENVISION) through MDA – controlling NTDs through what is generally regarded as cheap and effective drugs. However, some drug improvements are needed,[26] such as medicines effective for late phase of chronic disease for lymphatic filariasis. In addition, another five diseases are targeted by the London Declaration through intensified disease management and targeted by the WHO for elimination or eradication.[27]

Excluded from the London Declaration was dengue, which has been somewhat an oddity in the NTD group as a non-chronic disease affecting wealthier communities too – its contradictory status is explored in more depth in Chapter 4. Also excluded are six other diseases (buruli ulcer, cysticercosis/ taeniasis, echinococcosis, foodborne trematodiases, rabies, and yaws), treatable by antibiotics or animal/food management requiring public health measures in behaviour modifications and regulations. A variety of common tools exist to treat them, but they still remain persistent because systematic change is required. Therefore, the London Declaration focused on a more targeted 'tool-ready' list (and USAID even more so) where there is one easily deployable and effective measure of MDA.

In the earliest NTD report by the WHO (2004), 'tools for control' were a focus in developing new tools and refining of existing ones. Of the tools available, MDA was emphasised as "… safe, rapidly effective, and easy to administer in resource-poor settings, delivered by non-specialists, only once-yearly contact … major open-ended drug donations are making these tools available to all in need, as long as needed" (ibid., p. 56). For other diseases, the development was required of tools for use under difficult conditions and to improve safety and effectiveness. NTDs were thus evaluated on whether they are 'tool-ready' for public health interventions, depending on several questions, including 'What options are available for decision-making and implementation?' and 'What is the public health strategy and plan for action?'

Hotez and Pecoul (2010, p. 1) had previously outlined how 'tool-deficient' NTDs are as a group. They questioned whether NTDs had the correct tools available to them, including drugs, operational research on implementation, field-based diagnostics, health education for prevention, case detection and treatment, vector-control strategies, as well as improvements in water and sanitation. They made the point that all NTDs are tool-deficient in that tools exist to control, but the tools and implementation strategies have been "… suboptimal, incomplete, or inadequate to sustain elimination efforts … Consequently, substantial investments in R&D are urgently needed to develop new-generation control tools and strategies for their improved use and implementation" (ibid., pp. 2–3). What comes across is a 'mixed bag' of policy tools available for NTDs.

It is worth noting that the term 'policy tool' has lineage within the public policy literature – from the 1980s' and 1990s' policy design research to more current work on instrumentation through policy strategy and implementation (Howlett, 1991). A 'tools approach' by government is a popular means of intervention to move the focus away from impact to choice (Salamon & Lund, 1989). Gales and Lascoumes (2007) describe a policy tool as a 'micro device', paralleled in health policy with individual interventions for a disease. For NTDs, the language of tools becomes an essential part of talking about solutions as tools are linked to innovation, in the varied 'tool-kit' that is imagined. Some diseases are described as 'tool-ready', with appropriate innovations at hand, or 'tool-deficient' when innovation is lacking. These descriptions add a technical characterisation to the NTD policy problem where more innovation is equivalent to more tools to have at one's disposal.

Table 3.3 from the 2007 WHO report 'Global Plan to Combat Neglected Tropical Diseases 2008–2015', shows which NTDs are determined as tool-deficient or tool-ready. Here, tool-ready refers to interventions that can be used effectively to control or eliminate NTDs. The report refers to both NTDs and zoonoses, which may be why anthrax, brucellosis, and Japanese

Table 3.3 'Selected neglected tropical diseases and zoonoses to be addressed within the Global Plan'

Tool-ready diseases targeted for elimination or eradication by resolutions of the World Health Assembly and regional committees	Dracunculiasis Leprosy Lymphatic filariasis
Other tool-ready diseases	Anthroponotic leishmaniasis Blinding trachoma Cysticercosis Echinococcosis Rabies Schistosomiases Soil-transmitted helminthiasis Yaws
Tool-deficient diseases	Anthrax Brucellosis Buruli ulcer Chagas disease Dengue Human African trypanosomiasis Japanese encephalitis Leishmaniases Mycetoma, chromoblastomycosis and other deep mycoses Scabies and other ectoparasites Snakebite envenoming

(Adapted from WHO, 2007, p. 2 and Aya Pastrana et al., 2020)

encephalitis are included in this list. The table displays a relatively even split between NTDs that are tool-ready or deficient. Notedly, the new NTDs added in 2016 are all tool-deficient.

Excluded from the NTD group are diarrheal diseases,[28] as one of the "major tropical scourges but did not fit the 'insect-vector model' of the turn of the 20th century" (Worboys in Bynum & Porter, 2013, p. 522). Diarrheal diseases are WASH-related diseases, with WASH standing for inadequate water, sanitation, and hygiene, and some NTDs are included in this list.[29] Infections that cause diarrheal disease, for example, are cholera, dysentery, and typhoid. The lines drawn are blurred and have been based on historical contingencies.

Diarrheal diseases form part of an even broader list of 'infectious diseases of poverty', listed in Box 3.1. Malnutrition (or, more specifically, undernutrition or nutrient deficiency) does not make an entry into this list of infectious diseases of poverty. As a condition rather than a disease, it stands apart from the diseases of poverty, more often included under the banner of infant mortality and maternal mortality. What makes the NTD list and what does not (and indeed many other lists in public health categorisation) appear arbitrary in some ways. Therefore, Bhopal et al. question the usefulness of the NTD grouping, specifically with different organisations referring to various sub-categories (and even some additions) to the larger WHO grouping:

> Different stakeholders using the same term at any given time to encompass different diseases makes it difficult to set specific targets for control or to lobby for funding for NTDs as a group. Consequently, attention and funding are more aligned with the success of advocacy groups for

---

Box 3.1 List of infectious diseases of poverty

Infectious diseases of poverty (NTDs in bold)

- the Big Three, also called the three primary poverty-related diseases (PRDs): HIV, TB, and malaria diarrheal diseases
- *Salmonella* infections
- **helminth**
- bacterial pneumonia and meningitis
- **kinetoplastids** (human African trypanosomiasis, Chagas disease, and leishmaniasis)
- **dengue**

(Adapted from WHO, 2012)

individual diseases, with heavy reliance on pharmaceutical company donations, than to any objective criteria such as disease burden, attributed deaths or the need for new drugs, diagnostics and vaccines.

(2013, p. 1)

Their conclusion is that NTDs getting most attention exist in advocacy groups for individual diseases; and it appears, in referring to pharma donations, that they mean the five NTDs controlled through MDA. Individual diseases are still being lobbied for by deploying shorter lists from the WHO 20, through USAID or the London Declaration (with five other diseases).[30] Nick Kourgialis, from the NGO Helen Keller International, notes that it is an 'interesting discussion' whether to expand the range of diseases from the core five, citing pressure from organisations that represent the other diseases (interview with author, Kourgialis, 2016). However, he recognises the difficulty in trying to cover a large range of diseases, rather than focusing on a small group where public health tools are already available to address them, especially if eradication or elimination appears close:

> ... I mean, you know, there's been a lot of debate about that because there the question is whether we, detract from the current efforts to really finish the job to eliminate the diseases that we're focusing on now and there's a lot of investments that still need to be made and we don't want to lose that momentum or progress that's been achieved, because if we stop that, we kind of revert back to situation you had several years ago.
>
> (interview with author, Kourgialis, 2016)

The solution Bhopal et al. (2013) proposed was for the WHO to provide better leadership on NTDs, with a committee within the WHO Department of Control of Neglected Tropical Diseases to regularly review "... which new diseases should fall under the NTD umbrella" and how the "... successful branding technique of the NTDs can be magnified to deal with current and future neglected diseases" (ibid.). The proposal by Bhopal et al. has since been enacted. However what they did not highlight was the role of NGOs and their connection to scientist advocates and funders.

The major NGOs addressing NTDs span in their focus from treatment, funding, information, network, advocacy, along with sight charities and worm charities. Two scientist advocates later profiled have had a central involvement in almost half of the NGOs, and all of the NGOs apart from one (Deworm the World) are directly funded by the Gates Foundation. Peter Hotez is the president of one NGO (The Sabin Vaccine Institute), which spun out a key initiative (The Global Network). Alan Fenwick established an NGO (SCI), helped to found another (The End Fund), and is a partner of one more (Deworm the World). Incidentally, one of the founders of 'Deworm the World' was development economist Michael Kremer, who had written an influential paper on deworming three years before and more recently, 'Project Zero' by the Huffington Post, working with the Drugs for Neglected Diseases initiative (DNDi), was a year-long media and fundraising campaign funded by the Gates Foundation in 2016 to raise awareness around NTDs.

The diseases that these NGOs cover all vary. The question of which diseases fall under the umbrella of NTDs is an ongoing debate, reflecting the competitive and dynamic nature of global public health itself. Now that NTDs have policy currency, there is an obvious temptation to expand the grouping, matched by concerns about diluting the recognised branding and a need for coherence (an aspect of the WHO's strategic remit) in why diseases are included or not. This criteria about inclusion, prompted by Bhopal et al., was formalised in January 2016, at the 138th session of the WHO Executive Board, with the request for the Strategic and Technical Advisory Group (STAG) for Neglected Tropical Diseases to develop a "systematic, technically driven process for the adoption of additional diseases as NTDs" (WHO, 2016) (Box 3.2). The request led to a proposed criteria for classifying an NTD and process for review of the list of NTDs. The first point to note of this development is that the WHO's Regional Offices (ROs) already have their own lists "… which reflect diversity in geographical distribution of these diseases, and in some regions, they are considered the responsibility of other Departments" (ibid., pp. 1–2). The second point is on the grounds of what advocacy connected to being labelled an NTD can do:

> There are other conditions that could be classified as NTDs for the purpose of advocacy to motivate action or research for the development of new solutions in low resource settings. These are diseases or conditions that constitute important health issues in populations affected by poverty, but they do not fit the programmatic context as currently defined in WHO's HQ NTD Department's portfolio. Such diseases or conditions may however be included in the NTD list if, based on STAG recommendation, they can benefit from increased international attention in terms of advocacy, mobilization of resources for R&D and development of highly needed novel products and tools, or approaches for control or elimination.
>
> (ibid., p. 2)

Such a move demonstrates flexibility on the part of the WHO. The regional office for the Americas has two diseases not included in the WHO list: fascioliasis and hydatidosis. However, an overzealous reviewing process presents a danger, as noted already, brand if the diseases listed are widened or changed too frequently (Ozgediz & Riviello, 2008). The WHO also lists 'other neglected conditions', which have now constituted many of those added to the NTD list in 2016 – mycetoma, scabies, and snakebite (as well as podoconiosis included

---

Box 3.2 NTD disease conditions criteria for inclusion

Criteria for inclusion is given as:
  Disease conditions that:

1   disproportionately affect populations living in poverty and cause important morbidity and mortality – including stigma and discrimination – in such populations, justifying a global response.
2   primarily affect populations living in tropical and sub-tropical areas
3   are immediately amenable to broad control, elimination, or eradication by applying one or more of the five public health strategies adopted by the Department for Control of NTDs and/or are relatively neglected by research – i.e. resource allocation is not commensurate with the magnitude of the problem – when it comes to developing new diagnostics, medicines, and other control tools

(Adapted from the WHO, 2016)

---

briefly in 2011) were added but chronic suppurative otitis media (CSOM), nodding syndrome (NS), and strongyloidiasis were not (van de Sande et al., 2014). Krolewiecki and Nutman describe,

> From a public health perspective, the estimated size of the population affected and 'at risk' and its relationship to poverty and lack of adequate water and sanitation, puts strongyloidiasis squarely in the Neglected Tropical Disease (NTD) camp, although it is not currently incorporated in the World Health Organization's (WHO) strategy against STH.
> (Krolewiecki & Nutman, 2019, p. 2)

While sense needs to be made of the label, it is correct that caution should be applied in the use of the brand, especially if the end is in sight for some NTDs but not others, and that illusive end point is still yet to be reached.

Categories of inclusion or exclusion

What is included or not can tell us what importance we place on one thing over another. An often-cited definition of categories is by Goodwin:

> *In* so far as the coding scheme establishes an orientation toward the world, it constitutes a structure of intentionality whose proper locus is not the isolated, Cartesian mind, but a much larger organizational

system, one that is characteristically mediated through mundane bureaucratic documents such as forms.

(Goodwin in Bowker & Star, 1999, p. 65)

This description already points towards categorisation being more than a means of ordering, but as reflecting a way of looking at the world that is part of larger hierarchies and power structures. In 'Sorting Things out: Classification and Its Consequences', Bowker and Star cover an extensive array of case studies showing categories as historically situated artifacts with membership of certain groupings (1999, p. 285). Their contribution is in not theorising categories originating from the abstract sphere, but also as a product of communities of practice or the social world where certain activities are conducted together. They identify two sets of relationship that exist along the same trajectory: between people being given membership and objects being naturalised.

Bowker had also noted in earlier research that standardised representations are needed so that uncertainties or conflicts over meaning are overlooked, seen particularly through how "… medical classifications split up the world into useful categories" (1998, p. 187). Medicine may require more of an ordering that other areas of human endeavour and the effects are also deep and widespread. As Chaufan et al. observed relatedly that "… medical categories have the ability to create a social and moral order with a life of its own" (2012, p. 793).

Global campaigns and the 'Sustainable Development Goals'

Other diseases of poverty do have their own existing successful groupings, although neglect is also used as a characteristic. Cholera, dysentery, and typhoid have vaccinations to prevent illness and are closely associated with public-facing WASH campaigns, including initiatives such as the World Water Day, World Toilet Day, International Decade for Action 'Water for Life' 2005–2015 (UN Water n.d.). For NTDs there have also been global campaigns against individual diseases.

One of the first internationally coordinated initiatives addressing a NTD was the Onchocerciasis Control Programme (OCP), launched in 1974, with UN co-sponsorship (Liese, Rosenberg, & Schratz, 2010). OCP marked a high point for the WHO in the considerable success achieved. Accounts estimate 27,000 individuals were saved from going blind and 3 million children kept safe from onchocerciasis (Brown and Cueto in Parker & Sommer, 2010). The programme was further boosted by the efforts of the Carter Center since 1996 with the goal of eradication, followed by regional programmes in Africa and the Americas. Guinea worm (also pursued by the Carter Center since 1986), leprosy, and lymphatic filariasis were other notable global programmes,[31] all of which were essentially concerned with elimination and eradication. The

OCP came after the failure of the 'Global Malaria Eradication Programme', beginning in 1958 with the monumental task to eradicate malaria, but formally abandoned in 1969 (Feachem et al., 2010). The failure[32] may have had ongoing effects for the chosen methods of intervention for NTDs being drug-based rather than environmentally based, as the main method used to kill malaria-carrying mosquitos was chemical insecticide spraying of DDT.

The advocacy group 'Global Network for Neglected Tropical Diseases' was established by the Sabin Vaccine Institute in 2006, with Peter Hotez as the president and funding from the Bill & Melinda Gates Foundation (Global Network, n.d.). The Global Network runs the 'END7 campaign', launched in 2012 and focusing on the seven most common NTDs that represent 90% of the total NTD disease burden. The Global Network is different from the other campaigns discussed in that it is specifically an advocacy programme to raise the profile of NTDs with the public, philanthropists, policymakers, and politicians. Kari Stoever, who was the managing director, noted how single disease programmes had been operating independently, but the idea behind the work of the network was to group the diseases together (interview with author, Stoever, 2016). Similarly, one of the founding partners of the network was Helen Keller International, an NGO concerned specifically with blindness and malnutrition rather than NTDs generally. They found that, organisationally, they needed to change their strategy to adapt to the new NTD banner, with the approval of funding agencies such as USAID:

> ... there was not a lot of collaboration across program areas ... particularly by USAID were put under the umbrella of NTDs and, and there were five targeted diseases. So in order to pursue this integrated approach that was being you know, advocated by the USAID we had to add capacity to address these other diseases too, schistosomiasis and LF ... the integrated approach was really what was required and everybody was interested in the logic of that and the fact that these particular drugs that were focused on were tool-ready and there was really a strong case to be made for why the focus should be on these drugs, the commitment of the drug companies and other factors. And, you know, many of the people at the time had developed a very compelling case to Congress ... with the drug companies, convincing people that the real progress could be made in addressing these problems. So, for us in order to, to really be part of this effort we had to expand the scope of our activities.
>
> (interview with author, Kourgialis, 2016)

An integrated approach would allow Helen Keller to benefit from cost efficiencies in order to scale up efforts and also market the diseases better, further encouraged by the launch of an integrated NTD Control Program by USAID in 2006. The programme was the first 'global effort' to "... support country programs to integrate and scale up delivery of preventive chemotherapy for five targeted NTDs" (USAID's Neglected Tropical Disease Program, n.d.). It was based on donations of treatments, to fund the scale-up of treatment, working with disease-specific national control programmes to integrate MDA. Stoever describes the intentions of the network and how momentum was built:

> These programmes were operating quite robustly as single disease programs around the world but no one had put them all together in any single country and scaled it. So, the Global Network was really there to help facilitate that, bring resources, technical experts together to talk about how you would then take vertical programmes and create a horizontal approach and cost efficiency for that. We were awarded a grant from the Bill & Melinda Gates Foundation and that enabled us to set up a governance mechanism that would facilitate global scale-up. We were quite successful on the advocacy front, mostly in the US to begin with, which enabled countries to access new money to begin the harmonization process while the Global Network and partners advocated for more funding. This became a tipping point issue because we started to get access to private donors as well as other governments and foundations. We were featured at the Clinton Global Initiative three years in a row, and then went to Davos in 2009, so we were getting lot of exposure around the idea.
>
> (interview with author, Stoever, 2016)

The success of the Global Network was premised on the political connections forged, on platforms such as the Clinton Global Initiative Annual Meeting and annual World Economic forum in Davos. In the US, the connection with Congress – going right up to the President – was also crucial.

Political influence

Previously, Jimmy Carter (US President 1977–1981) had promoted onchocerciasis eradication after his presidency through his private foundation the Carter Center. However, NTDs would soon attract attention of a current president. Molyneux puts the connection with the Bush Whitehouse as being down to Stoever, who was the Managing Director of the Global Network (first interview with author, Molyneux, 2016). This involved liaising with the chief of staff on the idea of NTDs, when President George W. Bush (US President 2001–2009) went to Africa in 2008 and felt he had to make an announcement. Bush later announced $350m in funding for NTD treatment over five years, incorporating integrated NTD control through MDA and the scale-up of national programmes into the broader government global health agenda (Hotez & Goraleski, 2011). Barack Obama then expanded these programmes through his Global Health Initiative.

One NGO worker also spoke of the work of Hotez, advocating in Washington, tailoring his message to the audience, including the staff members of Senators in Congress:

> ... you have to understand your audience and so you really have to tailor the message to particular individuals and try to find whatever levers you have, that you have to switch to get them on board. And you need certain champions within different settings ... I remember, Peter Hotez visited the Hill and talked to some people from book parties where you know, very religious and talk about the Biblical plagues and try to make an association of these diseases with those, the old Biblical plagues and try to you know, create a connection in mind with the impact that these diseases were having. And, and so you use whatever you can to convey the importance of this and to link it to people's own concerns and attitudes. So yes, it doesn't take just one approach but you really have to lay out the information and provide an economic argument, certainly, but also talk about people's personal stories whenever you can.
>
> (interview with author, NGO worker, 2016)

In the UK, advocacy activity in political circles was matched, taking place there directly through scientist advocates. Stephen O'Brien, an MP and International Development Minister, was connected with Molyneux. Born in Tanzania, O'Brien founded and chaired an All Party Parliamentary Group on Malaria and Neglected Tropical Diseases in 2004 and pushed the agenda in the British Parliament. Molyneux viewed his "... sympathy for the cause having been born in Tanzania" (first interview with author, Molyneux, 2016). O'Brien argued on the value-for-money point that "(T)hose initiatives potentially have the most phenomenal value for money for the British people, as UK taxpayers, to be part of supporting" (House of Commons International Development Committee, 2012, ev. 27).

Another high-profile politician, Baroness Helene Hayman, became interested in NTDs through her son who was working with the Sabin Vaccine Institute. In 2011, after being Lord Speaker, she became Vice-Chair of the all-parliamentary group which set up to deal with malaria and had added NTDs to its remit in 2009. Through her political career, Baroness Hayman has seen the competition between diseases, in terms of "what is at the top of current political priorities, or public awareness" and is why she "... favours an evidence-led approach taking into account value for money where NTDs score strongly" (interview with author, Hayman, 2013). NTDs have become a bi-partisan, cross-party issue, and this wide political support has often relied on individual links to political decision-makers.

The political backdrop has also been important in determining the type of advocacy campaign pursued. As Chaufan et al. (2012) point out the importance of political opportunity structure of the US system for disease-specific research approach to funding. The UK system is also receptive to a 'disease-specific approach to funding' that emphasises disease categories to create a particular opportunity structure.

The Gates Foundation and technological solutionism

For philanthropic support, the major route for funding has been through the Bill & Melinda Gates Foundation. Gates set up his foundation following the model set out by Rockefeller, and also Carnegie, in large-scale phil-anthropy and applying business approaches (Solomon, 2011). Following this rationale, the Foundation has achieved a tremendous amount since inception in 1994 as a new global health actor. Spending around US$3 billion annually, it has "inaugurated an important new era of scientific commitment to global health predicaments" (Lancet, 2009). In deciding what areas of interest to concentrate on to have the greatest impact, the Gateses have said:

> (W)e concentrate on a few areas of giving so we can learn about the best approaches and have the greatest possible impact ... We choose these issues by asking: which problems affect the most people, and which have been neglected in the past.
>
> (ibid., p. 21)

Here, the concept of neglect played a central part in their strategy of choosing issues "to solve problems where no one else had stepped in", also informed by the scale of the problem and impact that was possible (ibid., p. 22). However, this line of thinking was not initially obvious. Kari Stoever recounts how the Bill & Melinda Gates Foundation was not interested in NTDs. Bill Gates was at first sceptical; but a few years later, he said to her that investing in NTDs was one of his proudest moments (interview with author, Stoever, 2016).

Gates has been described as "relentlessly rational" (Smith, 2015, p. 148). He had been a believer in Thomas Malthus, the 18/19th-century economist who warned about the growth of populations faster than the means of subsistence. The Gateses had begun with a Malthus-inspired approach when they began looking at public health in 1997 to focus on birth control:

> ... The logic was crisp and Bill Gates-friendly. Health = resources ÷ people. And since resources, as Gates noted, are relatively fixed, the answer lay in population control. Thus, vaccines made no sense to him: Why save kids only to consign them to life in overcrowded countries where they risked starving to death or being killed in civil war?
>
> (ibid.)

However, his thinking would change as he gathered more information about global health, seeing, for example, that if infant mortality rates dropped, people in developing countries had fewer children, as they would expect more children to survive into adulthood. Gates had been given an 82-book reading list in order to learn about international public health by William Foege, the former director of the CDC (Smith, 2015). He had stepped down from overseeing daily operations at Microsoft in 2008 to focus on the Foundation full time and had begun to become acquainted with NTDs. His favourite book from the reading list was the 1993 World Bank Report, and he described exactly what caught his attention:

> ... 'It was just a graph that had, you know, these twelve diseases that kill,' said Gates. These included leishmaniasis, schistosomiasis, trachoma – the list of leading scourges, preventable at low cost, whose names he'd also never seen before. 'I thought, 'This is 'bizarre',' Gates said. 'Why isn't this being covered?'...
>
> (Gates quoted by Smith, 2015, p. 145)

There was an appeal in the neglected aspect, as it gave the feeling of making a difference for the largest number, and measurement information about which diseases were a problem contributed to revealing this neglect:

> We couldn't believe it. You think in philanthropy that your dollars will just be marginal, because the really juicy obvious things will all have been taken. So you look at this stuff and we are like, wow! When somebody is saying to you we can save many lives for hundreds of dollars each, the answer has to be no, no, no. That would have already been done.
>
> (ibid.)

Large amounts of funding have been made available to NTDs as stated in 2021: "... To date, our team has committed more than US$1.02 billion in grants to organizations developing new tools and methods of delivery that make these tools widely available" (Gates Foundation, n.d.). It is 'new tools and methods' that are sought, as the Gates approach to global health problems also reflects a belief in the funding of science and technology to both see inequities and help address them (Solomon, 2011, p. 23).

How solutions are thought of is reflective of a technological 'solutionism' espoused by the writer Evgeny Morozov as the dominant ideology of everything needing to be fixed, but that we should rather be asking questions about the problem at hand. Solutionism, according to Morozov, is "(R)ecasting all complex social situations either as neatly defined problems with definite, computable solutions or as transparent and self-evident processes" for which he questions "both the means and the ends of Silicon Valley's latest quest to 'solve problems'" (Morozov, 2014, pp. 15–27). The technological aspect to solutionism puts forward a quick fix, rather than concentrating on more intel-lectually demanding reform (ibid., p. 34).

Little external scrutiny is directed towards this large-scale problem-solving. As Sridhar and Batniji (Lancet, 2009) have argued, there is not enough transparency or accountability to the Foundation's operation. Most grants go to organisations in high-income countries and multi-national company collaborators, and other important health programmes are distorted by the large grants (McCoy, 2009). Perhaps the most extensive critique has been by Linsey McGoey (2015b), in 'No Such Thing as a Free Gift', to catalogue some of the failings in the Gates approach to global health problems from the technology solutionism focus on vaccines and disease eradication that discount simpler, short-run solutions. As shown by the 'London Declaration' that Gates helped to orchestrate, NTDs are supported mainly through drug donation for those NTDs closest to elim-ination or eradication.

From drug donation to R&D

Aside from the sizeable donations by Gates primarily towards information collection[33] as well as advocacy,[34] the biggest donations have been drugs, and this has been generally well received and leveraged. Compared with other areas of public health, donations may be viewed more sceptically. For example, in 2016 the NGO 'Doctors without Borders' refused a one-million-dose dona-tion by Pfizer of the vaccine Prevnar 13 (PCV13) against pneumonia. In justi-fying the decision, this was a quote from MSF to *The Atlantic*:

> … 'I'm not absolutely against donations,' MSF's vaccine pharmacist Alain Alsahani told me by phone from Paris. In cases of neglected dis-ease where there is little or no market for a product, he explained, 'dona-tion becomes a more interesting option for some countries to get access. But in the case of PCV, that's not a solution at all, in any way'…
>
> (Hamblin, 2016)

The rationale in this case was that the donation did not justify the costs of delivering the vaccine and was not sustainable, nor large enough in number to include all who would need it. However, drug donations have formed the basis of advocacy for NTDs and have been built upon as a central interven-tion strategy, notably beginning with the first NTD donation by Merck for onchocerciasis in 1987 and led to pharma companies becoming involved in NTDs. Merck was the first company to action a large-scale donation of the drug ivermectin (marketed as Mectizan) through the 'Merck Mectizan Donation Program' (MDP) operating in sub-Saharan Africa, Latin America, and Yemen in the Middle East, constituting 33 of the 35 endemic countries (Sturchio, 2001).

Ivermectin had followed a successful and very profitable drug for deworming animals, which Merck scientists realised could have applications to humans. The subsequent donation was not a foregone conclusion, as Merck sought donor avenues to pay for the drug. After exhausting all options, the decision was made by the CEO to donate, in an unprecedented move for the size and reach of a pharma company donation. Many other drug donation programmes followed (Table 3.4), although it was not until the 2000s that these rose sharply in number, to also be extended and expanded with the London Declaration in 2012.

However, for every success story of drug donation, there is another of failure, highlighting the precarious nature of depending on free drugs (often at

Table 3.4 Drug donation for NTDs by date

Year	Disease and drug	Company
1987	**Onchocerciasis:** ivermectin	**Merck Sharp & Dohme (MSD)**
1997	**Lymphatic filariasis, STH:** albendazole	**GSK** (expansion 2010)
1998	**Trachoma:** Azithromycin	**Pfizer**
2000	**Leprosy:** multi-drug therapy (rifampicin, clofazimine, and dapsone in blister packs and loose clofazimine) and loose clofazimine in capsules since 2002	**Novartis**
2001	**HAT:** eflornithine, melarsoprol, and pentamidine	**Sanofi**[a] (until 2020)
2002	**HAT:** suramin	**Bayer** (until 2020)
2007	**Schistosomiasis:** praziquantel	**Merck**
2009	**HAT:** nifurtimox-eflornithine treatment combination (NEC)	**Bayer** (PPP with Sanofi to donate)
2009	**Fascioliasis (a foodborne trematodiases):** triclabendazole	**Novartis**
2011	**Visceral leishmaniasis: AmBisome**	**Gilead Sciences Inc.** (provided at discount since 1992)
2012	**Lymphatic filariasis:** diethylcarbamazine: DEC	**Eisai** (until 2020)
2012	**HAT and Chagas:** nifurtimox	**Bayer** (until 2021)
2012	**STHs:** mebendazole	**Johnson & Johnson** (until 2025)
2016	**Fascioliasis and paragonimiasis:** triclabendazole	**Novartis**
2017	**Visceral leishmaniasis:** liposomal amphotericin B	**Gilead Sciences Inc.** (until 2020)
2018	**Yaws:** azithromycin	**EMS** (Brazil)
2018	**HAT:** fexinidazole	**Sanofi**

a French company Aventis, which later became part of Sanofi, discontinued eflornithine production as it was not profitable; but Médecins Sans Frontières and the WHO persuaded the continued manufacture, leading to a comprehensive donation agreement (Potet, 2014).

(Compiled from WHO, 2012a and WHO, 2019)

the whim of pharma companies). One example is the drug eflornithine, used to treat HAT with fewer (of the quite terrible) side effects compared with previous drugs. Eflornithine had been registered in 1990 by the German pharma company Aventis, for treating cancer, and was subsequently adapted as a female facial hair reduction cream; but uptake and sales were low, so the company stopped production. This episode led, in the late 1990s, "to an outcry among public health specialists, who persuaded the company to reinstate production and, from 2001, to supply the drug for free in Africa" – a commitment that has continued after Aventis was acquired by Sanofi in 2004 (Jack, 2016).

Also despite commitments, the supply of drugs is not guaranteed – this is surprisingly so, even if responsibility is transferred to government. For example, 2012 saw a global shortage of the Chagas drug, benznidazole. Nine years previously, the technology and production of benznidazole had been transferred from the pharma company Roche to Lafepe, a Brazilian government pharmaceutical company (Manne et al., 2012, pp. 173–4). For a government-run operation, it could be expected that the drug would be produced without the limitations of profit-seeking; but production proved to be insufficient and inconsistent – a problem that mounted over the subsequent years.

This issue, on the whole, is an isolated one. An over-reliance on drug donation programmes may be especially problematic when production plants require investment and fail; companies go out of business or are acquired by other companies. Production plants run by pharmaceutical companies or governments may become a bigger problem in the future, with drug donations forming the basis for which the NTD advocacy case and policies have been built upon.

All donations typically form a type of public private partnership (PPP) for organisation and delivery. Drug donation PPPs have moved onto an R&D agenda where pharmaceutical companies seek to consciously develop drugs for NTDs, as companies still have to keep drugs affordable and innovate for new drugs sometimes through product development partnerships (PDPs) where collaboration centres on producing a new product. R&D projects are expanding to bring in new and improved drugs diagnostics and treatments. It was a criticism of both the TDR and GND that they did not directly produce new drugs, diagnostics, or vaccines. The TDR director John Reeder argued that doing this spun out from TDR supporting clinical trials:

> TDR identified the need for a new type of structure – a product development partnership (PDP). The Medicines for Malaria Venture, the Foundation for Innovative New Diagnostics and the Drugs for Neglected Diseases initiative were incubated within TDR and then spun out as independent entities.
>
> (International Innovation, 2014, p. 8)

By 2004, there were over 60 R&D projects,[35] according to the G-FINDER survey (Moran, Guzman, Burke, & Francisco, 2006). Of these, four new PPPs conducted nearly 75% of neglected disease drug development projects, including the Institute for OneWorld Health (iOWH), founded in 2000 to develop drugs, vaccines, and technologies for a range of diseases from malaria to diarrhea; the DNDi, founded in 2003 with a focus on the kinetoplastid diseases; and that same year, the Foundation for Innovative Diagnostics (FIND) was also established. DNDi has since had success with pharma company Sanofi in developing the first oral medication fexinidazole for HAT (Pelfrene et al., 2019) and FIND with pharma company Abbott has developed a rapid diagnostic test also for HAT (Hayashida et al., 2020). Other PPPs concentrate on specific diseases. Pharma company Novartis has an active dengue R&D programme at their 'Institute for Tropical Diseases' in Singapore (along with TB and Malaria), a leprosy donation programme and fund for R&D in Neglected Diseases (FRIND). Also, small independent pharma company Immtech has an R&D programme for Human African trypanosomiasis (HAT).

Stoever has expressed how PPPs have become standard models: "... to take a methodology and apply it for issue x ... what we learnt in the international space on global health is now being applied more and more to domestic issues at least in the US" (interview with author, Stoever, 2016). She also notes the change in role of pharma from principally providing drug donations: "today I think there's more leadership from the private sector, I like that pharma is embracing this more and is very proud of it" (ibid.).

Despite the drug dominance through NGOs and public discourse, the WHO has advocated an 'integrated approach' through national plans and a 'three-pronged' strategy of "... ensuring broader coverage with rapid impact interventions; strengthening vector control to reduce the transmission of several diseases; and improving surveillance and quality of care for diseases with limited control tools" (WHO, 2007, pp. 5–6). This 'three-pronged' strategy later became a 'five-pronged' strategy of:

- preventative chemotherapy
- innovative and intensified disease management
- vector ecology and management
- veterinary public-health services
- Provision of safe water, sanitation and hygiene

(WHO, 2015)

Still, drug interventions come first and tend to underpin much of the other activity, with R&D also supporting every stage.

Other sites of neglect

Big pharma is positioned as a main protagonist in why NTDs are neglected. However, often other sites of neglect such as the media are ignored. Conall Watson, an epidemiologist at the London School of Hygiene and Tropical

Medicine (LSHTM), spoke of the difference media attention makes to a health issue such as typhoid:

> Unless you can paint stuff as scientific breakthrough, I don't know how much of this stuff gets picked up in the mainstream press ... there are many ways to block typhoid transmission ... [other than the breakthroughs that are reported on].
>
> (interview with author, Watson, 2013)

He gave the example of typhoid, that in a policy-setting can be a difficult topic to broach, especially in terms of communication; and then the messages do not transfer well into the media:

> People don't really like to talk about poo on hands and using soap and that sort of stuff. It's much nicer to talk about clean water and new vaccinations, which I completely understand. And I suppose the other aspect that we don't often talk about is treatment and use of appropriate antibiotics.
>
> (interview with author, Watson, 2013)

The incremental work of the international research community and day-to-day typhoid treatment and control is not followed in the mainstream media, as it does not really fit with news agendas. News reporting is selective to scientific breakthrough and more attention-grabbing interventions, such as the use of innovation and technology in sanitation or vaccination. Therefore, media attention is difficult to sustain outside of more obvious news-grabbing headlines.

Balasegaram et al. (2008) surveyed NTDs in the English language media from 1 January 2003 to 1 June 2007 to conduct a content analysis of NTD media coverage. Qualitative interviews of the study revealed that American journalists struggled to cover global health issues as foreign news budgets had been slashed. They had further difficulty in reporting on relatively unknown diseases with limited information – finding it hard to get hold of spokespeople from the Gates Foundation or the WHO or stories from the field. The main findings of the study, which focused on leishmaniasis and trypanosomiasis, found the frames that were important and depicted the reality of the diseases; but, beyond descriptive frames, the popular focuses were:

- 'big pharma', where the industry was on the defensive or under pressure
- scientific developments from genetic research
- blood safety amidst the threat from Chagas (almost all US media articles).

> (Balasegaram et al., 2008, p. 4)

As might be expected, placing responsibility and blame for the problem of NTDs, with a focus on big pharma, is a major topic within the media. Science is positioned as a main solution for NTDs, and also making the news are threats to high-income countries as seen with the Chagas blood safety controversy of blood contaminated with the disease parasite. Seemingly absent are the global public health actors, a situation that may have changed more recently as we observe greater scrutiny of actors such as Gates (McGoey, 2015b; Lancet, 2009; Sridhar & Batniji, 2008).

Despite media-reporting only covering limited topics, the advocacy for NTDs has proved successful, a marker of which is in how NTDs have since been included in the Sustainable Development Goals (SDGs) for 2030. Dominic Haslam (2016), the director of policy and programme strategy at NGO Sightsavers, called the SDGs a "… once-in-a-generation chance to reframe NTDs within a more mainstream approach to health and development". Similarly, Molyneux, one of the scientist advocates, also reflected on what the SDGs meant as a sign of achievement and ongoing accountability of the global health community to NTDs:

> To have got NTDs included in the sustainable development goals for me was the most important achievement. Had they not been there, I would have thought that our efforts and advocacy would have failed. So, I really believe that was a big plus because they're embedded there semi-legally and so we can always point to them as being the targets.
>
> (second interview with author, Molyneux, 2016)

Exclusion from the MDGs in 2000 had set the ball rolling for NTD advocacy. Now the SDG, set out in 2015, specifically states: "By 2030 end the epidemics of AIDS, tuberculosis, malaria, and neglected tropical diseases and combat hepatitis, water-borne diseases, and other communicable diseases" (Target 3.3, Sustainable Development Knowledge Platform, n.d.). As there are 17 SDGs compared with the eight MDGs, the expanded agenda has been questioned. Haslam views the SDGs to be potentially unwieldy and undeliverable, but remains optimistic: "… the SDGs are a bold attempt to 'leave no one behind', a call I believe will see NTDs and other so-called 'lost causes' – and the millions of people they represent – finally brought out of the fringes of the development agenda" (2015). I summarise this chapter by putting into perspective this 'end point' of the SDGs with what has passed before, through a summary of the events and milestones that led to that point, and why they mattered.

Conclusion: beyond the SDGs

The chapter began with a discussion of two formative initiatives on tropical diseases starting in the 1970s. On one hand, the WHO's TDR initiative showed an early commitment to diseases of the poor but, ultimately, was not the conceptual origin for NTDs. As outlined, the reasons why were based in the institutional limitations of the WHO and the changing landscape of global health. On the other hand, the Rockefeller Foundation's GND initiative, while clearly having an influence in the naming of NTDs, had more relevance for NTDs in encouraging scientists to be interested in tropical diseases. Therefore, the GND was crucial in creating scientist advocates and in the future branding of NTDs. Next, I moved onto the key events in the policy development of NTDs, highlighting the two seemingly straightforward bookends with the MDGs in 2000 and the SDGs in 2015. The SDGs, in comparison to the earlier MDGs, include NTDs as a global policy priority and commitment. NTDs have now been confirmed as a mainstream concern through the same institutional setting that had previously left these diseases unacknowledged. The event milestones tracked this move from outsider to status quo through the MDGs to SDGs.

During the policy development of NTDs, organisations have used different lists of NTDs. The WHO has also provided distinctions based on pathogen and geography. The geographical distinction will be revisited in the final chapter as a way of understanding NTDs that challenge the donor and recipient country distinction on nationalist grounds. As I have shown, how the grouping of NTDs has changed reflects the state of public health globally. The WHO expanded their own grouping from 13 to 17 to 20, while *PLOS* expanded this group and the London Declaration and others shrank this group. The expansion and contraction is a reflection of the competitive nature of public health and the need to align disease to groups appropriately for policy reasons.

Still, the global health policy climate continues to evolve. There exists an optimism in the changing face of global public health, with a greater awareness of and interest in issues; and more people want to take a part: "I think with the emergence of Ebola … there are just more kids that want to study in this space. They don't necessarily all want to be scientists, but they want to work in global health" (interview with author, Stoever, 2016). Chapter 4 will further explore what this changing face by going back to the era of tropical diseases to review just how much has changed.

Notes

1   Defined as: "to treat with a scientific approach" (Merriam-Webster Dictionary).
2   Example, the Wellcome trust and Cancer Research UK.
3   Such as the National Institutes of Health (NIH) established in 1887 in the US and government funding of the Royal Society initiated in 1850 and 1913 when the Medical Research Committee (later the Medical Research Council) was established (Rosen, 1993; Kaiserfeld, 2013).
4   As was the closely related WHO group – the Division of Control of Tropical Diseases (CTD), established in 1990, which provided technical advice and assistance for endemic countries and jointly steered the TDR's applied field research. In 2007, CTD was incorporated into the HIV/AIDS, TB, and Malaria cluster (Lee & Fang, 2013).

5 Onchocerciasis.

6 When some governments disapproved of grant recipients (e.g. Burma), TDR made their case within the WHO that they had, "... the right to work with all Member States. Still, we had problems with some individuals. Some countries insisted that the government should nominate grant recipients. We refused, saying that it had to be about science not political favours" (Fleck, 2015, p. 293).

7 Others have explored the institutional settings of the WHO and the Rockefeller Foundation (Haynes, 1999), but research has not extended from tropical diseases to NTDs.

8 Run by the state of Geneva.

9 NTDs as a priority by the WHO in the goals of universal health coverage and essential health interventions can be seen in this statement by director Margaret Chan: "We are moving ahead towards achieving universal health coverage with essential health interventions for neglected tropical diseases, the ultimate expression of fairness" (WHO, 2013, p. vi).

10 Or rather the prospect of the green revolution to solve world hunger.

11 NTDs have often been affected by a focus on other scientific areas such as population growth and the green revolution. The later backlash against overuse of pesticides and insecticides in the concern for the environment had a detrimental effect on their use for vector control (Kinkela, 2011).

12 A major debate on whether to pursue the control and elimination of malaria was because of a knock-on effect on improved child mortality, worsening the problem of population growth. There was discussion among academics, policymakers, and in the media about the desirability of halting the malarial 'cull' which was a 30–40 per cent infant mortality rate to prevent population explosion in Asia and Africa (Fuller, 2015; J. N. Smith, 2015). China has relaxed its one child policy which, since 2015, is being formally phased out (BBC News, 2015); also, global fertility rates are dropping and even reverse population growth is seen in some countries such as Japan (Walsh, 2012).

13 'Mankind' was the common word at that time before the gender-neutral 'humankind' became more common. The GND had parallels then to the 'mankind' reference in the Rockefeller charter: "to promote the wellbeing of mankind throughout the world", a vision variously described as 'noble' (Keating, 2014) and less sympathetically as 'lofty' (Schanke, 2007).

14 Other uses of 'great' as a characterisation of tropical diseases included Ronald Ross in his autobiography, 'Memoirs of 1923', providing the subtitle "with a Full Account of the Great Malaria Problem and Its Solution" (Bynum & Porter, 2013, p. 562).

15 This interview was conducted with Dr Erman Sozudogru.

16 An earlier initial meeting in 2003 in Berlin was convened by the WHO and GTZ, on the 'Intensified control of neglected tropical diseases', defining a collective response against these diseases (WHO, 2004); although the 'Berlin Meeting' that most commentators refer to as the defining one was in 2005, which led to the creation of WHO Department for NTDs.

17 A popular definition from the late 1980s, coming from an influential public health inquiry by Acheson – the first since 1871 for the UK Government on 'Future Development to the Public Health Function', which used WHO categories as a basis for categorisation (Robotham & Frost, 2005).

18 Followed by an expanded 2006 paper, 'Incorporating a Rapid-Impact Package for Neglected Tropical Diseases with Programs for HIV/AIDS, Tuberculosis, and Malaria' (Hotez et al., 2006).
19 Can also be called a rapid impact package for five NTDs as soil-transmitted helminths (hookworm, trichuriasis, and ascariasis) are listed by the WHO together.
20 Called polyparasitism: "… concurrent infestation of a single host individual with two or more parasite species" (Zhou et al., 2010, p. 22).
21 He included six NTDs (Chagas disease, guinea worm, lymphatic filariasis, onchocerciasis, schistosomiases, and geohelminths) and also polio as his 'neglected' diseases.
22 As of 31 December 2015, from 2006, through annual donations from Warren Buffet (Gates Foundation, https://gatesfoundation.org/What-We-Do/Global-Health/Neglected-Tropical-Diseases, accessed 2/4/14).
23 The UK Government Department for International Development.
24 GlaxoSmithKline – a British pharma company.
25 For a breakdown of country classification by region (See United Nations Statistics Division, http://unstats.un.org/unsd/methods/m49/m49regin.htm#developed, accessed 2/4/14).
26 Also, vaccines and preventative drugs do not exist.
27 Dracunculiasis and leprosy are respectively close to eradication and elimination. Human African trypanosomiasis stands out in prevention and treatment, although elimination is viewed as possible. Similarly, Chagas disease and visceral leishmaniasis are viewed as controllable.
28 Infections of the intestinal tract, with rotavirus and E. coli bacteria the two most common etiological agents.
29 The WASH NTDs are soil-transmitted helminthiases, guinea worm, and schistosomiasis, all caused by parasitic worms except trachoma, caused by bacteria.
30 Onchocerciasis, schistosomiasis, trachoma, lymphatic filariasis, soil-transmitted helminthiasis (whipworm, hookworm, roundworm).
31 These were the Guinea Worm Eradication Program launched in 1980 at CDC; the Global Alliance for the Elimination of Leprosy launched in 1999; and the WHO's Global Programme to Eliminate Lymphatic Filariasis (GPELF) launched in 2000.
32 Malaria was eliminated in "Taiwan, much of the Caribbean, the Balkans, parts of northern Africa, the northern region of Australia, and a large swath of the South Pacific" (Gladwell, 2001).
33 Funding the G-FINDER and other reports.
34 Through the Global Network and organising the London Declaration.
35 Two malaria and TB projects counted in the 60 R&D projects (Moran, Guzman, Burke, & Francisco, 2006). They also include TDR, which they say, "has operated as a de-facto PPP since the mid-1970s" (ibid).

References

Acheson, D. 1988. "Public Health in England: The Report of the Committee of Inquiry into the Future Development to the Public Health Function." Department of Health and Social Security: Great Britain.

Aya Pastrana, N., D. Beran, C. Somerville, O. Heller, J. C. Correia & L. S. Suggs 2020. "The Process of Building the Priority of Neglected Tropical Diseases: A Global Policy Analysis." *PLoS Neglected Tropical Diseases* 14 (8): e0008498.

Balasegaram, M., S. Balasegaram, D. Malvy, & P. Millet. 2008. "Neglected Diseases in the News: A Content Analysis of Recent International Media Coverage Focussing on Leishmaniasis and Trypanosomiasis." *PLoS Neglected Tropical Diseases* 2 (5): e234. https://doi.org/10.1371/journal.pntd.0000234.

BBC News. 2015. "China to End One-Child Policy and Allow Two." *BBC*, October 29, 2015. https://bbc.com/news/world-asia-34665539.

Bhopal, A., T. Callender, A. F. Knox, & S. Regmi. 2013. "Strength in Numbers? Grouping, Fund Allocation and Coordination amongst the Neglected Tropical Diseases." *Journal of Global Health* 3 (2): 020302. https://doi.org/10.7189/jogh.03.020302.

Birn, A. -E., E. Fee, A.-E. Birn, M. Cueto, J. Farley, E. Fee, S. Hewa, & S. Palmer. 2013. "The Rockefeller Foundation and the International Health Agenda." *The Lancet* 381 (9878): 1618–19. https://doi.org/10.1016/S0140-6736(13)61013-2.

Borowy, I. 2009. *Coming to Terms with World Health: The League of Nations Health Organisation, 1921–1946.* Peter Lang. https://books.google.fr/books?hl=en&lr=&id=KuXv6zC09nMC&oi=fnd&pg=PA7&dq=League+of+Nations+Health+Organization+(LNHO)+has+been+modelled+on+the+Rockefeller+Foundation&ots=Qh3fliXKv3&sig=6UL2Qsh2Yc56e-mpgmgWp91iRPU&redir_esc=y#v=onepage&q=League of Nations.

Bowker, G. C. 1998. "The Kindness of Strangers: Kinds and Politics in Classification Systems." *Library Trends* 47 (2): 255–93.

Bowker, G. C., & S. Leigh Star. 1999. *Sorting Things out: Classification and Its Consequences.* MIT Press.

Bulletin of the World Health Organization. 2007. "Applying Science to the Diseases of Poverty: The Bulletin Interview with Dr Robert Ridley." *Bulletin of the World Health Organization* 85 (7): 501–68. https://who.int/bulletin/volumes/85/7/07-100707/en/.

Bynum, W. F., & R. Porter. 2013. *Companion Encyclopedia of the History of Medicine.* Routledge.

Chaufan, C., B. Hollister, J. Nazareno, & P. Fox. 2012. "Medical Ideology as a Double-Edged Sword: The Politics of Cure and Care in the Making of Alzheimer's Disease." *Social Science & Medicine* 74 (5): 788–95. https://doi.org/10.1016/j.socscimed.2011.10.033.

Chen, L. C. 2014. "China Medical Board: A Century of Rockefeller Health Philanthropy." *The Lancet* 384 (9945): 717–19. https://doi.org/10.1016/S0140-6736(14)60965-X.

Conrad, P., & Barker, K. K. 2010. "The Social Construction of Illness: Key Insights and Policy Implications." *Journal of Health and Social Behavior* 51 (1_suppl): S67–S79.

Cotton, R. 2015. "Neglected Tropical Diseases: Challenges for the Post-2015 Development Era." *PLOS ECR Community*, February 8, 2015. http://blogs.plos.org/thestudentblog/2015/01/01/neglected-tropical-diseases-challenges-post-2015-development-era/.

Farley, J. 2004. *To Cast out Disease: A History of the International Health Division of the Rockefeller Foundation (1913–1951).* Oxford University Press.

Feachem, R. G. A., A. A. Phillips, J. Hwang, C. Cotter, B. Wielgosz, B. M. Greenwood, O. Sabot, et al. 2010. "Shrinking the Malaria Map: Progress and Prospects." *The Lancet* 376 (9752): 1566–78. https://doi.org/10.1016/S0140-6736(10)61270-6.

Fleck, F. 2015. "Former TDR Director Ade Lucas Profiled in WHO Bulletin." *WHO Bulletin.*

Fudenberg, H. H. 1983. *Biomedical Institutions, Biomedical Funding, and Public Policy.* Plenum Press.

"Gates Foundation." n.d. Accessed May 15, 2016. https://gatesfoundation.org/What-We-Do/Global-Health/Neglected-Tropical-Diseases.

Genève Internationale. 2014. "Interview with John Reeder, Director of TDR, UN Flagship Programme for Research and Scientific Collaboration on Diseases of Poverty," Accessed May 21, 2014. https://geneve-int.ch/interview-john-reeder-director-tdr-un-flagship-programme-research-and-scientific-collaboration-disea.

Gillam, S. 2008. "Is the Declaration of Alma Ata Still Relevant to Primary Health Care?" *BMJ (Clinical Research Ed.)* 336 (7643): 536–8. https://doi.org/10.1136/bmj.39469.432118.AD.

Gladwell, M. 2001. "The Mosquito Killer." *The New Yorker*, July 2, 2001. http://gladwell.com/the-mosquito-killer/.

Global Network. n.d. "Global Network." Accessed September 14, 2015. https://globalnetwork.org/.

Haberman, C. 2015. "The Unrealized Horrors of Population Explosion." *The New York Times*, May 31, 2015. https://nytimes.com/2015/06/01/us/the-unrealized-horrors-of-population-explosion.html?_r=0.

Hamblin, J. 2016. "Doctors Without Borders Refuses Vaccines from Pfizer." The Atlantic. 2016. https://theatlantic.com/health/archive/2016/10/doctors-with-borders/503786/.

Haslam, D. 2015. "Will the SDGs Be the Last Hope for Lost Causes?" *The Guardian: Global Development Professionals Network*, February 20, 2015. https://theguardian.com/global-development-professionals-network/2015/feb/20/will-the-sdgs-be-the-last-hope-for-lost-causes.

———. 2016. "Is This a Turning Point for Neglected Tropical Diseases?" The Huffington Post. 2016. https://huffingtonpost.co.uk/dominic-haslam/tropical-disease_b_7559636.html.

Hayashida, K., P. Nambala, N. Van Reet, P. Büscher, M. Kawai, M. M. Mutengo, J. Musaya, B. Namangala, C. Sugimoto, & J. Yamagishi, 2020. "Development of a Bio-Inkjet Printed LAMP Test Kit for Detecting Human African Trypanosomiasis." *PLoS Neglected Tropical Diseases* 14 (10): e0008753.

Haynes, D. M. 1999. "The Social Production of Metropolitan Expertise in Tropical Diseases: The Imperial State, Colonial Service and the Tropical Diseases Research Fund." *Science, Technology & Society* 4 (2): 205–38.

Holt, F., S. J. Gillam, & J. M. Ngondi. 2012. "Improving Access to Medicines for Neglected Tropical Diseases in Developing Countries: Lessons from Three Emerging Economies." *PLoS Neglected Tropical Diseases* 6 (2): e1390. https://doi.org/10.1371/journal.pntd.0001390.

Hotez, P. J., M. Elena Bottazzi, E. Dumonteil, J. G. Valenzuela, S. Kamhawi, J. Ortega, S. P. de Leon Rosales, M. B. Cravioto, & R. Tapia-Conyer. 2012. "Texas and Mexico: Sharing a Legacy of Poverty and Neglected Tropical Diseases."

PLoS Neglected Tropical Diseases 6 (3): e1497. https://doi.org/10.1371/journal.pntd.0001497.

Hotez, P. J., & K. A. Goraleski. 2011. "Neglected Tropical Diseases and the 2012 US Presidential Election." *PLoS Neglected Tropical Diseases* 5 (11): e1431. https://doi.org/10.1371/journal.pntd.0001431.

Hotez, P. J., D. H. Molyneux, A. Fenwick, E. Ottesen, S. E. Sachs, & J. D. Sachs. 2006. "Incorporating a Rapid-Impact Package for Neglected Tropical Diseases with Programs for HIV/AIDS, Tuberculosis, and Malaria." *PLoS Medicine* 3 (5): e102. https://doi.org/10.1371/journal.pmed.0030102.

Hotez, P. J., & B. Pecoul. 2010. "'Manifesto' for Advancing the Control and Elimination of Neglected Tropical Diseases." *PLoS Neglected Tropical Diseases* 4 (5): e718. https://doi.org/10.1371/journal.pntd.0000718.

House of Commons International Development Committee. 2012. *South Sudan: Prospects for Peace and Development*. The Stationery Office. https://books.google.com/books?id=dN7A3h-CuToC&pgis=1.

Howlett, M. 1991. "Policy Instruments, Policy Styles, and Policy Implementation. National Approaches to Theories of Instrument Choice." *Policy Studies Journal* 19 (2): 1–21. https://doi.org/10.1111/j.1541-0072.1991.tb01878.x.

Jack, A. 2016. "Waking up to Sleeping Sickness." *Financial Times*, April 29, 2016. https://ft.com/intl/cms/s/0/1c1eba64-0cc6-11e6-ad80-67655613c2d6.html.

Kaiserfeld, T. 2013. "Why New Hybrid Organizations Are Formed: Historical Perspectives on Epistemic and Academic Drift." *Minerva* 51 (2): 171–94. https://doi.org/10.1007/s11024-013-9226-x.

Keating, C. 2014. "Ken Warren and the Rockefeller Foundation's Great Neglected Diseases Network, 1978–1988: The Transformation of Tropical and Global Medicine." *Molecular Medicine* 20: S24–S30. https://doi.org/10.2119/molmed.2014.00221.

Kenny, K. E. 2015. "The Biopolitics of Global Health: Life and Death in Neoliberal Time." *Journal of Sociology* 51 (1): 9–27. https://doi.org/10.1177/1440783314562313.

Kinkela, D. 2011. *DDT and the American Century: Global Health, Environmental Politics, and the Pesticide That Changed the World*. University of North Carolina Press. https://books.google.com/books?id=9iYrOPezt7IC&pgis=1.

Kreier, J. P. 2014. *Malaria: Immunology and Immunization*. Elsevier Science. https://books.google.com/books?id=mJniBQAAQBAJ&pgis=1.

Krolewiecki, A., & T. B. Nutman. 2019. "Strongyloidiasis: A Neglected Tropical Disease." *Infectious Disease Clinics of North America* 33 (1): 135–51. https://doi.org/10.1016/j.idc.2018.10.006.

Lammie, P. J., J. F. Lindo, W. Evan Secor, J. Vasquez, S. K. Ault, & M. L. Eberhard. 2007. "Eliminating Lymphatic Filariasis, Onchocerciasis, and Schistosomiasis from the Americas: Breaking a Historical Legacy of Slavery." Edited by C. H. King. *PLoS Neglected Tropical Diseases* 1 (2): e71. https://doi.org/10.1371/journal.pntd.0000071.

Lancet. 2009. "What Has the Gates Foundation Done for Global Health?" *The Lancet* 373 (9675): 1577. https://doi.org/10.1016/S0140-6736(09)60885-0.

Lascoumes, P., & P. Le Gales. 2007. "Understanding Public Policy through Its Instruments? From the Nature of Instruments to the Sociology of Public Policy Instrumentation." *Governance* 20 (1): 1–21. https://doi.org/10.1111/j.1468-0491.2007.00342.x.

Lee, K., & J. Fang. 2013. *Historical Dictionary of the World Health Organization*. Rowman & Littlefield. https://books.google.com/books?id=9zCEmpopjG0C&pgis=1.

Liese, B. H., & L. Schubert. 2009. "Official Development Assistance for Health–How Neglected Are Neglected Tropical Diseases? An Analysis of Health Financing." *International Health* 1 (2): 141–7. https://doi.org/10.1016/j.inhe.2009.08.004.

Liese, B., M. Rosenberg, & A. Schratz. 2010. "Programmes, Partnerships, and Governance for Elimination and Control of Neglected Tropical Diseases." *The Lancet* 375 (9708): 67–76. https://doi.org/10.1016/S0140-6736(09)61749-9.

Lucas, A. O. 2013. "Research and Training in Tropical Diseases." *Interdisciplinary Science Reviews* 3 (3): 220–4. https://doi.org/10.1179/030801878791925958.

Manne, J., C. S. Snively, M. Z. Levy, & M. R. Reich. 2012. "Supply Chain Problems for Chagas Disease Treatment." *The Lancet. Infectious Diseases* 12 (3): 173–5. https://doi.org/10.1016/S1473-3099(12)70001-4.

Manson, P. 1898. "Tropical Diseases: A Manual of the Diseases of Warm Climates." London, [&c.]: Cassell and Company, Limited (Electronic Resource London School of Hygiene and Tropical Medicine). 1898. https://archive.org/details/b21356038.

McCarthy, M. 2002. "A Brief History of the World Health Organization." *The Lancet* 360 (9340): 1111–12. https://doi.org/10.1016/S0140-6736(02)11244-X.

McCoy, D. 2009. "The Giants of Philanthropy." *The Guardian*, April 5, 2009. https://theguardian.com/commentisfree/2009/aug/05/gates-foundation-health-policy.

McGoey, L. 2015a. *No Such Thing as a Free Gift: The Gates Foundation and the Price of Philanthropy*. https://books.google.ch/books/about/No_Such_Thing_as_a_Free_Gift.html?id=nSQgrgEACAAJ&pgis=1.

———. 2015b. "Would the Gates Foundation Do More Good without Bill?" *The Guardian*, November 3, 2015. https://theguardian.com/commentisfree/2015/nov/03/gates-foundation-without-bill-philanthropic.

Merriam-Webster Dictionary. n.d. "Definition of Scientize." https://merriam-webster.com/dictionary/scientize.

Molyneux, D. H. 2004. "'Neglected' Diseases but Unrecognised Successes–Challenges and Opportunities for Infectious Disease Control." *The Lancet* 364 (9431): 380–3. https://doi.org/10.1016/S0140-6736(04)16728-7.

———. 2008. "Combating the 'Other Diseases' of MDG 6: Changing the Paradigm to Achieve Equity and Poverty Reduction?" *Transactions of the Royal Society of Tropical Medicine and Hygiene* 102 (6): 509–19. https://doi.org/10.1016/j.trstmh.2008.02.024.

Molyneux, D. H., P. J. Hotez, & A. Fenwick. 2005. "'Rapid-Impact Interventions': How a Policy of Integrated Control for Africa's Neglected Tropical Diseases Could Benefit the Poor." *PLoS Medicine* 2 (11): e336. https://doi.org/10.1371/journal.pmed.0020336.

Moran, M., J. Guzman, M. A. Burke, & A. L. de Francisco. 2006. "Drug R&D for Neglected Diseases by Public-Private Partnerships: Are Public Funds Appropriately Distributed?" *Monitoring Financial Flows for Health Research 2005: Behind the Global Numbers*. Edited by M. A. Burke and A. L. de Francisco. Global Forum for Health Research. https://georgeinstitute.org.au/publications/drug-rd-for-neglected-diseases-by-public-private-partnerships-are-public-funds.

Morel, C. M., T. Acharya, D. Broun, A. Dangi, C. Elias, N. K. Ganguly, C. A. Gardner, et al. 2005. "Health Innovation Networks to Help Developing Countries Address Neglected Diseases." *Science* 309 (5733): 401–4. https://doi.org/10.1126/science.1115538.

Morozov, E. 2014. *To Save Everything, Click Here: Technology, Solutionism and the Urge to Fix Problems That Don't Exist*. Penguin Books.

Ozgediz, D., & R. Riviello. 2008. "The 'Other' Neglected Diseases in Global Public Health: Surgical Conditions in Sub-Saharan Africa." *PLoS Medicine* 5 (6): e121. https://doi.org/10.1371/journal.pmed.0050121.

Parker, R., & M. Sommer. 2010. *Routledge Handbook of Global Public Health*. Routledge. https://books.google.com/books?id=RIqsAgAAQBAJ&pgis=1.

Pelfrene, E., M. H. A., N. Ntamabyaliro, V. Nambasa, F. V. Ventura, N. Nagercoil, & M. Cavaleri, 2019. "The European Medicines Agency's Scientific Opinion on Oral Fexinidazole for Human African Trypanosomiasis." *PLoS Neglected Tropical Diseases* 13 (6): e0007381.

PLOS Neglected Tropical Diseases. n.d. "Journal Information." Accessed January 28, 2016. http://journals.plos.org/plosntds/s/journal-information.

Potet, J. 2014. "Neglected Tropical Diseases and Access to Medicines: Time to Think beyond Drug Donations." | *The Lancet Global Health Blog*, April 1, 2014. http://globalhealth.thelancet.com/2014/04/01/neglected-tropical-diseases-and-access-medicines-time-think-beyond-drug-donations.

Reeder, J. 2014. "World Health Organization Special Programme for Research and Training in Tropical Disease." *International Innovation*. https://international innovation.com/40-years-of-fighting-diseases-of-poverty/.

Relman, E., & D. Choffnes. 2011. The Causes and Impacts of Neglected Tropical and Zoonotic Diseases: Opportunities for Integrated Intervention Strategies: Workshop Summary *The National Academies Press. Forum on Microbial Threats; Institute of Medicine*. https://nap.edu/catalog/13087/the-causes-and-impacts-of-neglected-tropical-and-zoonotic-diseases.

Remme, J. H. F., E. Blas, L. Chitsulo, P. M. P. Desjeux, H. D. Engers, Thomas P. Kanyok, Jane F. Kengeya Kayondo, et al. 2002. "Strategic Emphases for Tropical Diseases Research: A TDR Perspective." *Trends in Parasitology* 18 (10): 421–6. https://doi.org/10.1016/S1471-4922(02)02387-5.

Robotham, A., & M. Frost. 2005. *Health Visiting: Specialist Community Public Health Nursing*. Elsevier Health Sciences. https://books.google.com/books?id=64--p0LAVYEC&pgis=1.

Rosen, G. 1993. *A History of Public Health*. Johns Hopkins University Press.

Rosenberg, C. E., & J. L. Golden. 1992. *Framing Disease: Studies in Cultural History*. Rutgers University Press. https://books.google.com/books?hl=en&lr=&id=agi08b NtBwgC&pgis=1.

Salamon, L. M., & M. S. Lund. 1989. *Beyond Privatization: The Tools of Government Action*. The Urban Institute. https://books.google.com/books?hl=en&lr=&id=BXI 2nGfivJQC&pgis=1.

Sande, W. W. J. van de, E. S. Maghoub, A. H. Fahal, M. Goodfellow, O. Welsh, & E. Zijlstra. 2014. "The Mycetoma Knowledge Gap: Identification of Research Priorities." *PLoS Neglected Tropical Diseases* 8 (3): e2667. https://doi.org/10.1371/journal.pntd.0002667.

Savioli, L., A. Montresor, & A. F. Gabrielli. 2011. "Neglected Tropical Diseases: The Development of a Brand with No Copyright: A Shift from a Disease-Centred to a

Tool Centred Strategic Approach." National Academies Press. https://ncbi.nlm.nih. gov/books/NBK62524/.

Schanke, R. A. 2007. *Angels in the American Theater: Patrons, Patronage, and Philanthropy.* SIU Press. https://books.google.com/books?id=MEDLIJdtFnEC &pgis=1.

Schneider, A., & H. Ingram. 1990. "Behavioral Assumptions of Policy Tools." *Journal of Politics* 52 (2): 510–29. https://doi.org/10.2307/2131904.

Smith, J. N. 2015. *Epic Measures: One Doctor. Seven Billion Patients.* https://books. google.ch/books/about/Epic_Measures.html?id=EvqEoAEACAAJ& pgis=1.

Solomon, L. D. 2011. *Tech Billionaires: Reshaping Philanthropy in a Quest for a Better World.* Transaction Publishers. https://books.google.com/books?id=jmkdbrhlfK8C &pgis=1.

Sridhar, D., & R. Batniji. 2008. "Misfinancing Global Health: A Case for Transparency in Disbursements and Decision Making." *The Lancet* 372 (9644): 1185–91. https:// doi.org/10.1016/S0140-6736(08)61485-3.

Sturchio, J. L. 2001. "The Case of Ivermectin: Lessons and Implications for Improving Access to Care and Treatment in Developing Countries." *Community Eye Health / International Centre for Eye Health* 14 (38): 22–3. https://pubmedcentral.nih.gov/ articlerender.fcgi?artid=1705916&tool=pmcentrez&rendertype=abstract.

Sustainable Development Knowledge Platform. n.d. "Sustainable Development Goals." United Nations. Accessed March 31, 2016. https://sustainabledevelopment. un.org/?menu=1300.

The Official PLOS Blog. n.d. "Announcing PLoS Neglected Tropical Diseases." Accessed May 1, 2016. http://blogs.plos.org/plos/2006/09/announcing-plos-neglected-tropical-diseases/.

U.S. Congress Office of Technology Assessment. 1985. *Status of Biomedical Research and Related Technology for Tropical Diseases: Summary.* DIANE Publishing. https://books.google.com/books?id=bzlXhfZ-w2AC&pgis=1.

UN Water. n.d. "UN Water: Campaigns." Accessed April 19, 2016. https://unwater. org/campaigns/world-water-day/en/.

United Nations Statistics Division. n.d. "Standard Country and Area Codes Classifications (M49)." Accessed April 19, 2016. http://unstats.un.org/unsd/ methods/m49/m49regin.htm#developed.

Uniting to Combat NTDs. 2014. "Delivering on Promises and Driving Progress: The Second Report on Uniting to Combat NTDs." 2014. http://unitingtocombatntds. org/sites/default/files/document/NTD_report_04102014_v4_singles.pdf.

USAID's Neglected Tropical Disease Program. n.d. "Newsroom, Voices from the Field, Uganda." Accessed April 20, 2016. https://neglecteddiseases.gov/newsroom/ voices_from_the_field/uganda_trachoma.html.

Walsh, B. 2012. "Why Declining Birthrates Are Good for the Planet." *Time*, March 14, 2012. http://science.time.com/2012/03/14/population-studies-birth-rates-are-declining-for-the-earth-and-a-lot-of-people-thats-not-a-bad-thing/.

WHO. 2004. "Intensified Control of Neglected Diseases: Report of an International Workshop Berlin, 10–12 December 2003." http://apps.who.int/iris/bitstream/10665/ 68529/1/WHO_CDS_CPE_CEE_2004.45.pdf?ua=1.

———. 2005. "Strategic and Technical Meeting on Intensified Control of Neglected Tropical Diseases: A Renewed Effort to Combat Entrenched Communicable Diseases of the Poor." *Report of an International Workshop Berlin, 18–20 April 2005.* http://apps.who.int/iris/bitstream/10665/69297/1/WHO_CDS_NTD_2006.1_ eng.pdf.

———. 2007. "Global Plan to Combat Neglected Tropical Diseases 2008–2015." http://apps.who.int/iris/bitstream/10665/69708/1/WHO_CDS_NTD_2007.3_eng. pdf.

———. 2012a. "Accelerating Work to Overcome the Global Impact of Neglected Tropical Diseases: A Roadmap for Implementation: Executive Summary." Geneva: World Health Organization. http://apps.who.int//iris/handle/10665/70809.

———. 2012b. "Global Report for Research on Infectious Diseases of Poverty." World Health Organization. https://who.int/tdr/publications/global_report/en/.

———. 2013. "Sustaining the Drive to Overcome the Global Impact of Neglected Tropical Diseases: Second WHO Report on Neglected Tropical Diseases." World Health Organization. https://who.int/neglected_diseases/9789241564540/en/.

———. 2015. "First WHO report on neglected tropical diseases: Working to overcome the global impact of neglected tropical diseases." World Health Organization. Retrieved from https://who.int/neglected_diseases/2010report/en/.

———. 2016. "Report of the WHO Strategic and Technical Advisory Group for Neglected Tropical Diseases." 2016. https://who.int/neglected_diseases/NTD_STAG_report_2015.pdf.

———. 2019. "Contribution of Pharmaceutical Companies to the Control of Neglected Tropical Diseases." World Health Organization. 2019. https://who.int/neglected_diseases/pharma_contribution/en/.

WHO TDR-CTD. 1990. "WHO Division of Control of Tropical Diseases (CTD)." WHO. 1990. https://ciesin.org/docs/001-614/001-614.html.

Zhou, X. -N., R. Berguist, R. Olveda, & J. Utzinger. 2010. *Important Helminth Infections in Southeast Asia: Diversity and Potential for Control and Elimination, Part 2.* Academic Press. https://books.google.com/books?id=MWOI7z7m1M8C&pgis=1.

Zhou, X. -N., S. Wayling, & R. Bergquist. 2010. "Concepts in Research Capabilities Strengthening Positive Experiences of Network Approaches by TDR in the People's Republic of China and Eastern Asia." *Advances in Parasitology* 73: 1–19. https://doi.org/10.1016/S0065-308X(10)73001-3.

Part II

Becoming un-neglected

Chapter 4

The transition of tropical diseases

Tropical and neglected categories

I ask what is tropical, both in terms of historical and geographic location – a line of enquiry that has precedence in exploring the social embeddedness of disease and is central to challenging colonial accounts (Anderson, 1996; Bewell, 2003; Blaut, 2012). In exploring the tropical, there is a vast literature on the role of tropical medicine in support of the colonial project (Amaral, 2008; Arnold, 1996; Chakrabarti, 2013, 2017; McNeil Jr., 2012; Neill, 2012; D'Arcy & Worthen, 1999) and a relatively more recent literature on the policy developments for neglected tropical diseases (NTDs) (Hotez et al., 2014; Molyneux et al., 2005; Parker, Allen, & Hastings, 2008). These two literatures rarely meet. Therefore, tropical diseases become diseases of the past, a matter of historical record, and are only to be understood through the context of colonialism and empire. NTDs are not mature enough, as a disease grouping to have a historical account and have not received an extensive social science gaze. NTDs are a fledging field for social science research, but to understand these diseases in any depth also requires a connection with the past.

The tropical category will be explored through (1) a brief colonial as well as post-colonial history; and (2) current geography, where the chronic characterisation of disease and a concept of blue marble health in viewing disease distribution becomes relevant. The specialism of tropical medicine has been of research interest across what is now an extensive historical, sociological, geographical, political science, and anthropological literature (LSHTM, 2014), but has been varyingly attributed to diseases thought to be common or more specific to the tropics and sub-tropical regions. Beginning with the origins of tropical medicine, this chapter first identifies what is 'tropical', followed by what is 'neglected' in NTDs.

What is 'tropical'?

There are two parts to the tropical categorisation – the place of 'tropical' in history and the place in geography. Of course, these overlap but can be thought of in terms of colonial history and current geography. Loomba describes colonialism as the practice of "the conquest and control of other people's land and goods" (2005, p. 20).[1] By the time of the Treaty of Paris in 1776,[2] Spain's dominance as a European power had been broken, giving way to a new era of English colonialism. Over a decade later, 1787 is identified by Stepan as when the phrase 'tropical disease' was first used in English medical work for illnesses associated with hot climates (2001, p. 17). Stepan goes on to say: "Almost by definition, tropical medicine was a colonial medicine" (ibid., p. 28). It existed, as Ring describes, to play "... a pivotal role in negotiating the relationship between the colonised and the colonisers since it constituted a powerful discourse of authority and modernity" (2003, p. 5). Post-empire, the field remains in what has been called "... a residual category, synonymous with the additional requirements of imperial medical practice" (Worboys in Bynum & Porter, 2013, p. 512).

Tropical medicine has been a problem-based specialism based on the problem of undertaking medicine practice in the tropical colonies, rather than a bio-medical basis to the disease grouping (e.g. based on pathogen or geography) (Lemaine et al., 1976). The British physician Patrick Manson was founding director of the London School of Hygiene and Tropical Medicine (LSHTM), a training ground for physicians to treat British colonial administrators as well as others who worked in Britain's tropical empire. He was largely behind creating the specialism of tropical medicine and his book, 'Manson's Tropical Diseases: A Manual of the Diseases of Warm Climates' (1898)[3] was definitive in the construction of the grouping, listing a catalogue of 65 infections or diseases from the minor 'prickly heat' to the more serious malaria and yellow fever.[4] Today, definitions of NTDs do still differ, depending on the source, with the most definitive list of 20 NTDs given by the WHO. Manson, at the turn of the 20th century, listed 10 of the 20 NTDs listed by the WHO (see Table 4.1) drawn from his much larger list of 65.[5]

Of the diseases listed by the WHO that were not included by Manson in his list, two appear to have predated discovery (Chagas disease in 1909 and Buruli ulcer, which was only described a year before Manson's 1898 publication). In the case of chromoblastomycosis, it was in 1922 that the term was coined to refer to the disease (de Brito & Bittencourt, 2018). Other diseases would have been familiar to Europeans and so not seen as especially tropical: taeniasis or cysticercosis may have been the reason why pork was considered impure to some societies (Del Brutto & García, 2015), scabies was a skin infection associated with poverty (McCarthy et al., 2004), snakebite was more common, and trachoma was associated with armies and was being controlled in Europe (Mohammadpour et al., 2016). Rabies now joins the NTD group clustering in the tropics but, at the time, was persistent in central Europe for much of the 19th century and is likely to be why Manson did not list it as tropical (Bourhy et al., 2010).

Table 4.1 Comparing WHO list of NTDs to Manson's list of tropical diseases

'20 WHO'	'Manson 11'
1. Buruli ulcer	
2. Chagas disease	
3. Dengue and chikungunya	x
4. Dracunculiasis (guinea-worm disease)	x
5. Echinococcosis	
6. Foodborne trematodiases	
7. Human African trypanosomiasis (sleeping sickness)	x
8. Leishmaniasis	x
9. Leprosy (Hansen's disease)	x
10. Lymphatic filariasis	x
11. Mycetoma, chromoblastomycosis and other deep mycoses	x
12. Onchocerciasis (river blindness)	x
13. Rabies	
14. Scabies and other ectoparasites	
15. Schistosomiasis	x
16. Snakebite envenoming	
17. Soil-transmitted helminthiases	x
18. Taeniasis/cysticercosis	
19. Trachoma	
20. Yaws (endemic treponematosis)	x

(Compiled from Manson, 1898; WHO, 2016a)

Many diseases listed by Manson are now not classified as NTDs, are more rarely seen (plague) if ever, today (goundou). Others have had vaccines, which has meant more targeted intervention campaigns (yellow fever, Japanese encephalitis, typhoid) or easily treatable mild conditions (heat-stroke, prickly heat, boils). Another large section of diseases includes archaic medical terms, being more symptom than disease (craw-craw) or holding commonalities with NTDs but not the specific type now viewed as a problem. For example, dog tapeworm (distomum heterophytes) being listed by Manson, rather than pig tapeworm (taenia solium), the leading cause of preventable epilepsy. Finally, there are still the time-persistent diseases associated with poverty that were once pandemic and now cluster in the tropics: malaria, cholera, and dysentery. Malaria has since joined the Big Three high-mortality global disease grouping amassing a large amount of attention and funding alongside HIV/AIDS and TB (Molyneux, 2008). Cholera and dysentery are typically called 'diseases of poverty' and are 'diarrheal related', but are of most concern during humanitarian emergencies when they can become epidemic (Parker & Sommer, 2010).

The relationship between disease categorisation, scientific discovery, and economic development certainly has not been static. Despite the persistence of some diseases, there has been an evolving conception of disease as a result of scientific progress and economic development, which extends to the category of tropical disease challenging preconceived notions. Robert Desowitz, a tropical disease specialist and popular science writer, noted: "Well, these diseases that we call 'typically tropical' have been as American as the heart attack" (quoted by Killheffer, 1997). Even at the time of creation, the category posed difficulties. Manson "… acknowledged that the term tropical diseases was 'more convenient than accurate' …" (ibid.). However, this grouping of convenience has had consequences in inheriting the geographical assumptions of colonial medicine (Bewell, 2003, p. 36). The associated meanings of 'tropical' have included 'climatic handicaps', 'inertia', 'degeneration', 'primordial', and 'treacherous', demarking "… sharp moral and topographical distinctions between tropical and temperate climates" (Ring, 2003, pp. 1–2). These derogatory meanings have led to scientists and policymakers – especially from the tropics – to dispute and challenge the tropical disease characterisation.

A prominent example is Afrânio Peixoto, who was the Chair of Hygiene at Rio de Janeiro's Faculty of Medicine and a vocal objector to the designation because of the denotation of biogeographic curse or fate of climate being responsible for disease. In the early 20th century, he argued that tropical medicine:

> … reinforced the prejudices associated[6] with climatic determinism and old stereotypes created by Europeans who 'defamed' the 'torrid' countries as insalubrious lands unsuited to civilization. Peixoto declared that there were no tropical diseases since there were no climatic diseases.
>
> (Kropf, 2011, p.18)

Some later objections were more confrontational. This is an account from Desowitz working on tropical medicine in the 1960s:

> In 1962, when Indonesia's dictator, Sukarno, was in flower, I attended a meeting of the Southeast Asian Ministers of Education (Secretariat Tropical Medicine Project). The representative from Indonesia opened the session by hotly proclaiming that there was no such thing as 'tropical' medicine; it was a colonial term of denigration (the implication being that the whites were hygienic and the natives unsanitary) …
>
> (Desowitz, 1997, p. 11)

This reaction was not without reason as a sanitary survey was often 'an integral part' of British colonial medicine; and, if the question of a nation's authority and modernity are at stake, it is not surprising that there is a need to create distance from what had been seen as diseases of domination and backwardness or an uncivilised past (Ring, 2003, p. 3). However, dealing with these diseases also formed a part of medical practice. As Hotta wrote in 1989, "bacteriology, parasitology, dietetics, sanitary hygiene, etc. derived from, or evolved in parallel with tropical medicine" (Hen, 1989, p. 2).

The inter-connectiveness of colonialism with science and medicine is a reason behind an intellectual movement of the postcolonial world to criticise science and medicine as an instrument of Western hegemony through a cultural specificity of scientific truths (see Adams, 1998). One reaction has been to oppose universalist objectivity but, in the case of tropical disease, we have seen almost the reverse happening. Harding (1993) describes a 'strategy of universalization' in rejecting the concept of tropical diseases. Here, in reaction to the relativist version of disease through tropical places and people, was the attachment of disease to a universal idea. This idea was reflected at a later date through an example taken from the late 1990s, in the suggestion that a new term was used:

> when the organisation of European Schools of Tropical Medicine (TropMed Europe) met in Addis Ababa in 1997, they were persuaded by African Colleagues that the term 'tropical medicine' still had patronising colonial overtones and should be replaced by 'international medicine' although that decision was never implemented.
>
> (Eddleston et al., 2008)

The history of tropical medicine has, therefore, involved the interplay between universality and particularity. The tropical regions were viewed as particular with their climate of heat and moisture being deemed inhospitable to white people. The formulation of 'germ theory' hailed an era of 'new tropical medicine' (Lemaine et al., 1976, pp. 84–5). A generalised 'European approach' could be applied because the causes of disease were germs, so that scientific knowledge could defeat disease and allow for tropical colonialisation. Post-World War II, tropical medicine would be influenced by other scientific disciplines: "fundamental biology, chemistry, physics, etc." leading to experimental and clinical medicine (Hen, 1989, p. 2).

The end of colonialism left open a number of possible redirections to take tropical medicine. What approach would be taken – universalist or particularist? Would it be understood as region-based or pathogen-based? Would expertise rely on on-the-ground public health experience or the introduction of new scientific disciplines? Post-empire, it looked as if that the name 'tropical medicine' might be dropped altogether.

Tropical re-relevance

Evidently the change to 'international medicine' did not happen (at least not on a wholesale basis)[7] and so a persisting concern amongst tropical disease advocates was whether the term 'tropical disease' lacked relevance. The association with colonialism would be a driver for a renaming, to escape the framing that arises from the aims and visions of a colonial past. The new term 'NTDs' has appeared to displace some of these previous colonial connotations. However, it seems this might go full circle. Bill Gates, for example, has spoken of his hopes for the neglected to be gone with, still referencing the tropical: "Maybe as the decade goes on, people will wonder if these should be called neglected diseases. Maybe as the milestones go on, we will call them just tropical diseases" (Gates quoted by Boseley, 2012). Hotez and Musgrove have similarly said: "Lymphatic filariasis, onchocerciasis, schistosomiasis, soil-transmitted helminth infections, and trachoma are starting to lose the 'N' from NTD" (2009, p. 1700). The message being sent out is that tropical has been a point of tension and, after the renaming, it turns into something ostensibly more neutral. However, the intention behind the renaming is that it will serve a purpose and no longer be used at some point.

What is left is an interesting conflict that arises when calling something 'neglected'. To refer to something as neglected is a labelling act, an evocation for it to not be so. The diseases are called neglected so that, at a point in the future, they will be no longer. Thus, it is only a temporary term if the hopes of advocates are realised. However, neglect will exist on a scale, and the diseases within will be relatively, more or less, neglected. This is an impreciseness and definitional quality that is not based on biology or other material descriptors like 'tropical' and something that some in the scientific community were initially opposed to. For example, Simon Croft, a Professor of Parasitology at the London School of Hygiene and Tropical Medicine (LSHTM), highlighted that 'neglect' was a labelling concept that could cause difficulty in the division made across biological categories:

> If you start labeling things as neglected, I understand it from an advocacy point of view but … some people don't start looking across the board at the discipline, strategy. Whatever you're doing on infectious diseases it's the same principles … you don't want to fragment things too much … it's great for advocacy to raise the profile and get lots of publicity.
>
> (interview with author, Simon Croft, 2014)

Current geography

The second positioning of 'tropical' is in geography. The geographical assignment, as pointed out by Manson in establishing the tropical medicine speciality (Manson, 1898), is more convenient than accurate, to assign diseases a locality within tropical or semi-tropical regions. Boundaries are stretched and blurred as to which countries count as 'tropical'. Stepan notes, Algeria was considered medically tropical in the late 19th century, even though it was not in a literal geographic sense. 'Tropical' was more than a geographic concept and "… signified a place of racial otherness to the temperate world" (2001). Diseases that counted as 'tropical' did not easily fit classification, and it is inaccurate to think of these diseases as a foreign 'other'. Manson noted at the turn of the 20th century that "… a volume on diseases peculiar to the tropics would occupy six pages or so" (Worboys in Bynum & Porter, 2013, p. 512).

Tropical diseases are certainly more fluid than would be expected, and their geography is constantly shifting. What we have called tropical diseases in the past – malaria, for example – have existed in the southern US states and went as far north as Boston and even Montreal (Conn, 2011). This is not ancient history, either. Until the beginning of the 20th century, the mosquito-borne diseases malaria and yellow fever were a serious problem in the southern US farming regions (Desowitz, 1991). One out of every eight citizens of Memphis, Tennessee was dying of yellow fever before eradication in 1949 (Conn, 2011). A 'pin-up' calendar for US troops was made by The Center for Disease Control (CDC), which was founded during World War II as the Office of Malaria Control (see Figure 4.1). The agency was charged with running mosquito abatement programmes and publicity campaigns, especially around military bases, until eradication in the US in 1951.

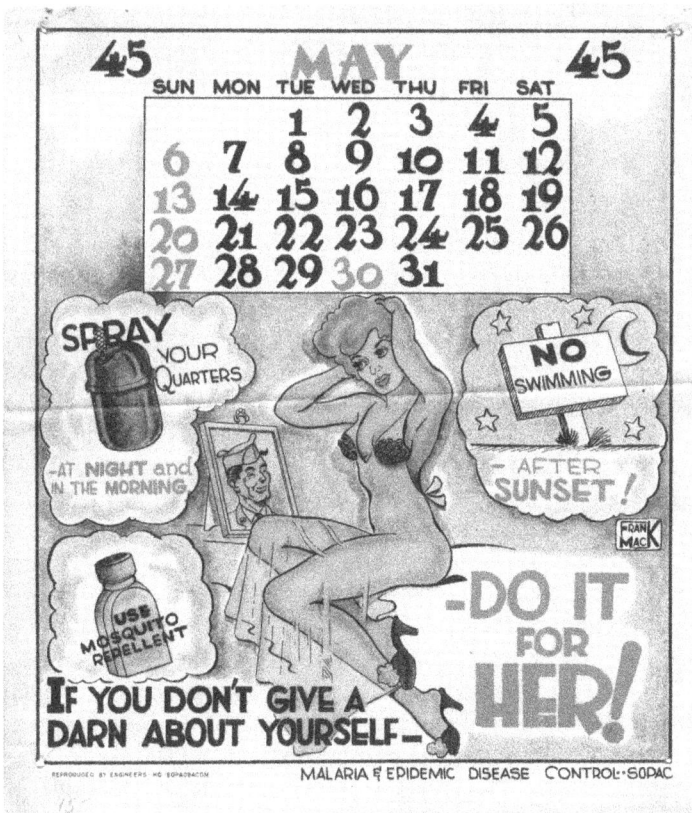

Figure 4.1 'Pin-up' calendar poster by Office of Malaria Control.

(NPR.com 'How the U.S. Stopped Malaria, One Cartoon at a Time', 2012)

In Italy, malaria[8] was called the 'Italian National Disease'. By 1904, the country had begun a 'crusade against malaria', involving the state, local government, and medical profession through mass quinine purchase,[9] a quinine tax of employers and landowners, support of the Italian Red Cross and rural health stations to administer the treatment (Snowden, 2006). The idea of nationhood was prevalent throughout, as Prime Minister Sonnino stated in 1910:

> ... the fight against the terrible scourge of malaria constitutes an important economic, social, and public health interest for our nation ... No effort must be neglected. Only the contribution of everyone, no one excepted, and the unremitting employment of every available means ... will make it possible to achieve significant and lasting results.

> (ibid., p. 61)

Thus, now forgotten, tropical diseases have been significant in the histories and feature of now high-income countries, reflecting their culture and society.[10] Forgetting has been a part of neglect; it is an inadvertent neglect of a past once known, but can also be deliberate by ignoring the past.

Challenging geographic classification: chronically tropical

Today, yellow fever and malaria no longer tend to be classed as NTDs. This brings the discussion to diseases that could be thought of as tropical diseases but are not. HIV/AIDS and TB, although having high incidence rates in the tropics, are now not viewed as especially tropical. Kamat (2013) explains the shift in perceptions for malaria between 2001 and 2013: "... malaria is no longer indexed as a 'tropical disease'; it is placed on par with HIV/AIDS and tuberculosis as a global killer, at least discursively, demanding renewed attention and enormous resources" (p. 221). The change was partly a result of the Millennium Development Goals (MDGs), agreed by all member countries at the UN and leading development institutions.

These developments propelled malaria, HIV/AIDS, and TB as targets for global attention in 2000, rather than being consigned to the tropics, to be global killers, because of the scale of deaths, and so the sixth goal out of the eight poverty reduction goals was "... to combat AIDS, malaria, and other diseases".[11] TB was later to be included in this grouping, through the 'Global Fund to Fight AIDS, TB and Malaria'. This example shows how other disease constructs form an identity (the Big Three) giving rise to disease identities in relation, so that the 'other diseases' in the MDGs became NTDs. Outliers to NTDs can be learnt from, in yellow fever and dengue fever, which have been argued to be included or not.

Yellow fever

Yellow fever is not seen as a particularly neglected disease, although it is certainly tropical, with the virus endemic across the tropical area of Africa and Latin America covering 44 countries (with estimated deaths of up to 60,000 a year in 2020) and the potential to cause significant disruption to global trade and travel (WHO, n.d.). An effective vaccine exists and control programmes have been successful in the past. Therefore, the existence of these interventions, as well as yellow fever not being a chronic disease, appear to be why it is excluded. However, rabies is included when an effective vaccine exists, and it is not a chronic disease either. Thus it is likely that rabies is included as a tropical zoonotic[12] disease, which better fits the NTD profile; and vaccination programmes are expensive, especially when better animal management can also work, and it affects the rural poor living in remote areas (Bourhy et al., 2010). Therefore, a number of the characteristics of rabies are a very good fit. However, some do identify yellow fever as an NTD, on the basis of lack of research:

> Yellow fever is truly a neglected tropical disease ... Even though it continues to cause fatality, it remains understudied. While it is true there is a highly effective vaccine, it remains extremely challenging to get comprehensive vaccine coverage in sub-Saharan Africa and Latin America. Moreover, the vaccine works well if you are between one and 55 years old. It is not safe for babies or the elderly, who could develop yellow fever from the vaccine.
>
> (Pittalwala, 2014)

It is also likely not to have been included in the NTD grouping as an arbovirus (arthropod-borne virus found in mosquitoes, ticks, flies transmitting pathogens to humans), while NTDs are more dominated by parasitic, protozoal, and bacterial diseases. This exclusion on the grounds of pathogen has led to some scholars, such as LaBeaud, making the case for the inclusion of arboviruses.[13] The list goes on for diseases that scientists argue should be listed, and that have since been included:

> ... snakebite is a disease that kills 100,000 a year so should be on list, I think there's a momentum there, now Sanofi has stopped making the anti-venom and Africa are in serious trouble ... so I'm really a great advocate for snakebite.
>
> (first interview with author, Molyneux, 2016)

Subsequently, snakebite has been included, but not yellow fever. Conversely, arguments attest for other diseases to be taken off the list, as shown next with dengue.

Dengue

Dengue is an example of the changing perception of NTDs as it is an arbo-virus and was a late addition to the NTD list in 2010 (Hotez, 2011). As yellow fever incidence rates are rising where regular vaccine programmes have not been implemented, there may be future inclusion. What appeared to justify inclusion of dengue is the lack of an effective treatment until recently, when a vaccine was developed and its presence in the tropics that is rising "… both in space and time, becoming less and less seasonal, and occurring in more parts of the world" (Conn, 2011). Therefore, previous lack of research and intervention tools are crucial – an increased and unacknowledged burden – as Cameron Simmons argues: "(D)engue is neglected in the sense that the true scale of the disease burden is poorly understood and certainly underestimated" (Regnier, 2012a).

However, it does raise questions being an arbovirus, not chronic, and not being a disease strongly related with poverty. Participants at a 2011 workshop, held by the Institute of Medicine in Washington, questioned the inclusion of dengue. The following is an account from the workshop, where "(T)here was considerable controversy as to whether or not Dengue is an NTD", with some arguing it is an emerging (acute febrile) illness, rather than a chronic debili-tating one and "therefore does not fit the NTD model" (Relman & Choffnes, 2011). The 'chronic disease nature' is a feature of neglect (covered in the next section) compared with other infectious diseases. Chronic infectious diseases more rarely cause 'explosive outbreaks', making them less visible and not well exported to higher-income countries, even though they are communicable, so are not seen as a threat (Relman & Choffnes, 2011, p. 17). Therefore, the idea of diseases being 'tropical' is in part due to containment in lower-income countries. An example of an explosive outbreak that might be thought of as a tropical disease in 2014 was Ebola. As another arbovirus, it is classed as an emerging disease,[14] even while being found in tropical regions and some arguing it has been neglected.

Dengue has been described as a semi-commercial disease,[15] in that some aspects of treatment development in the past have not been commercially viable, but other avenues such as vaccines have potentially high rewards if targeted towards richer consumers and countries. Sanofi has invested €1.3bn in their dengue vaccine Dengvaxia and expected to recoup their costs, with analysts predicting it could become "the world's best-selling vaccine with revenues of €1bn a year" (Ward, 2014). If pharmaceutical companies can successfully target consumers and governments in high-income countries such as Singapore and middle-income countries (Brazil and China), they will see profits – especially as dengue does not affect the poor dispropor-tionately. For example, the middle class was the predominant group affected during the epidemic in Dhaka, Bangladesh, and upper social classes had higher seroprevalence rates[16] in Fortaleza and San Luis epidemics in Brazil (Guha-Sapir & Schimmer, 2005, p. 5). However, Dengvaxia has since been embroiled with controversy because of deaths that were linked with the vaccine in the Philippines (Gubler & Halstead, 2019).

Mulligan et al. (2015), through a systematic review of the research literature, found that the relationship between dengue and poverty is not well established. They also questioned, in an earlier paper, what the consequences were in "public health policies that construe dengue as a disease of poverty" and whether there are more appropriate policies for dengue in middle or upper-middle class communities than the current construction as an NTD (Mulligan et al., 2012, p. 409). While it is evident that global strategies for dengue in poor communities become adapted to local conditions, Mulligan et al. also make the political observation that:

> For the WHO, reconsidering dengue-poverty connections may also mean revisiting the question of why dengue is a neglected tropical disease, shifting responsibility for dengue from the characteristics of poor populations and communities themselves to the political decisions that have resulted in under-investment in this rapidly spreading infectious disease.
>
> (ibid., p. 415–6)

They point towards the decisions of rapidly developing countries where better urban planning is needed, alongside a consideration of public health policies related to new living situations (ibid.). As Gavin Screaton describes, "(D)engue is predominantly a disease of urbanisation … It poses major challenges to healthcare systems in developing countries because of its epidemic potential causing explosive outbreaks in some major cities" (Regnier, 2012a).

The inconsistencies for dengue with other NTDs form part of a larger debate about disease categorisation. The inclusion in the NTD list appears to have been driven by concern about incidence rates and epidemics after the disease was made an international public health priority by the WHO in 2002. There is no other obvious group for dengue to have gone under (apart from perhaps 're-emerging diseases') and so NTDs provide a helpful banner. However, the arguments made by both Mulligan et al. and the participants at the Institute of Medicine Workshop expose the consequences of categorisation. On a national level, a dengue strategy characterised by poverty avoids political questions about urbanisation and development, as well as not being well suited to local needs. While on a global level, there is a raised concern for dengue, in the potential for crossing borders from tropical regions and posing an epidemic threat.

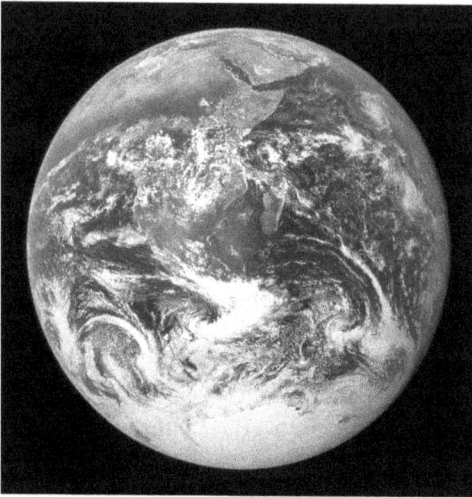

Figure 4.2 'Blue Marble Earth'.

(NASA https://nasa.gov/, accessed 10 December 2016)

Blue marble health

What, then, are the consequences of over-focusing on the tropical and not addressing other considerations? The contradiction between the geographically tropical imagination of these diseases and what some argue as more accurate characterisation by poverty (whether in a tropical country or otherwise) is the concept espoused by Peter Hotez called 'blue marble health'. The idea of blue marble health is a blurring of health between higher- and lower-income countries so that within G20 countries (an international forum for governments and central bank governors consisting of 19 countries and the European Union) we also see NTDs. Hotez makes the argument that NTDs still exist within poor communities in higher-income countries. Diseases do not affect countries homogenously; instead, there are local inequalities and disparities. There exist many layers of inequality in global health, and this point is made in reference to the photograph of Earth taken by the Apollo 17 astronauts to portray a view of the world as being one whole, looking like a blue glass marble (see Figure 4.2). The extreme poor live among the wealthy and disproportionately suffer from the world's NTDs, as Hotez describes:

> ... we're finding paradoxically that more than half the neglected diseases are occurring among the G20 countries but they are occurring in areas of poverty in those countries. Places like Southern Mexico or Northern Argentina or Northeastern Brazil or in Indonesia ... countries have the

ability to afford treatments for neglected tropical diseases so it calls on the G20 countries to take responsibility for their own diseases, and, I'll just say that we are often now finding this hidden burden of neglected tropical.

(interview with author, Hotez, 2014)

To summarise, it is already evident that the tropical category causes some tension, as there may be some diseases that are tropical but not neglected, and vice versa. The disputes about where inclusion lines are drawn signifies how tropical disease is related to a particular idea of disease that goes beyond even the geographical location and historical categories. From here, the next question is the neglected categorisation, and this too is far from straightforward.

What is 'neglected'?

The 'neglected' category is arguably even more contentious. It is significant to attribute a socio-political categorisation to diseases. Similar terms that refer to the place of diseases in society and politics are 'diseases of poverty' such as diarrhoea and pneumonia or 'lifestyle diseases' caused by obesity and smoking. The influence of epidemiology can be seen to have had a profound effect through concern for the distribution and (social) determinants of health (Raphael, 2006). However, these disease categories can be problematic in terms of the values and choices applied, whether for individuals and/or societies.

What is the difference between a disease of poverty and a lifestyle disease? Ironically, today, a disease such as scurvy could be placed in the category of lifestyle diseases (Dobson, 2015), caused by a particular way of living. In the past, the disease was seen to be due to limited scientific knowledge to know it was caused by a lack of nutrition, but now that the knowledge is available and it is preventable, responsibility and blame are passed to the patient. Both groups of diseases, whether due to poverty or lifestyle, may focus blame on the individual or society, although lifestyle diseases connote more of an element of choice when compared with poverty. Thus, the argument might follow that the state should not fund treatment.

Similarly, a disease of poverty connotes stigma; so again, there might be social consequences for being within this category.[17] At the Institute for Tropical Medicine in São Paulo, the doctors praised media campaigns addressing the taboo of TB (interview with author, Scientist at Institute for Tropical Medicine, 2014). Over time, a reaction to NTDs has been stigma and social marginalisation, documented by sociological research on the cultural meaning of stigmatised illness. 'Stigmatised illness' was a category used by Erving Goffman, Zachary Gussow, and George Tracy in the 1960s for leprosy, and subsequently for epilepsy, cancer, HIV/AIDS, and sexually trans-mitted diseases (STDs) (Conrad & Barker, 2010, p. S69). They identify how illnesses become stigmatised, the impacts, the ways individuals and groups manage stigma, and how stigma can change over time.

Leprosy is one stigmatised NTD, but many others have similar features in terms of disfigurement and disability (e.g. visceral leishmaniasis and trachoma). Stigma perpetuates the hidden nature of disease that happens to the poor, their voices unheard, sickness and deaths not acknowledged, diagnosed, or treated. It is a "... lack of political voice among those afflicted by neglected tropical diseases ... neglect diseases of neglected people" (Relman & Choffnes, 2011, p. 17). Therefore, the neglected description can be argued to be an acknowledgement of the already socio-political nature of disease, in how stigma leaves patients hidden and voiceless.

Definitions of neglect

The NTD group as outlined by the WHO relies on a 'new conceptual framework' based on commonalities decided by the organisation and set out in the first report on NTDs in 2010. As the WHO points out in the report, these are a medically diverse set of diseases (2010) and thus need justification for grouping. These commonalities offer insight into the policy rationale for grouping NTDs:

- a proxy for poverty and disadvantage
- affect populations with low visibility and little political voice
- do not travel widely
- cause stigma and discrimination, especially of girls and women
- have an important impact on morbidity and mortality
- are relatively neglected by research
- can be controlled, prevented, and possibly eliminated using effective and feasible solutions

Others have followed suit in considering the WHO list of commonalities and providing further detail. Relman and Choffnes have drawn on NTD experts (Hotez & Pecoul, 2010) to give some explanation behind the WHO common-alities (Box 4.1). The authors place further emphasis on how 'underdevelop-ment' is exacerbated; contrast between those affected and decision-makers in capital cities; the effect of stigma and discrimination for women's marriage prospects and vulnerability to abuse or abandonment; and NTDs not travel-ling easily, so are not a threat to inhabitants of high-income countries. This list appears to draw out the unequal aspects of NTDs with dualities between the developed and underdeveloped; decision-makers and the voiceless; women and men; and high-income inhabitants and low-income inhabitants.

Box 4.1 NTDs and their common features

The NTDs are quite a diverse and heterogeneous group of diseases. However, they share a number of common features:

1 *the hallmark of poverty and underdevelopment*

The most striking common feature of the NTDs is that they affect almost exclusively poor and marginalised populations.

2 *diseases of non-decision-makers*

Affected populations often live in remote rural area, in conflict zones, or in urban slums and have little political voice. They cannot readily influence administrative and governmental decisions that affect their health and often seem to have no constituency that speaks on their behalf. Diseases associated with rural poverty may have little impact on decision-makers in capital cities.

3 *association with stigma and discrimination, especially of women*

Many NTDs produce disfigurement and disability, leading to stigma and social discrimination. Their impact disproportionally affects women, whose marriage prospects may diminish or who may be left vulnerable to abuse and abandonment

4 *not travelling*

Unlike influenza, HIV/AIDS, malaria, and, to a lesser extent, tuberculosis, NTDs generally do not travel and seem to present little threat to inhabitants of high-income countries. Rather, the distribution of NTDs is restricted by climate, and its effect on the distribution of vectors and reservoir hosts there appears to be little risk of transmission beyond the tropics.

(Adapted from Relman & Choffnes, 2011)

These commonality lists have since evolved into a more affirmative 'criteria for inclusion' discussed in the last chapter, with the STAG group for Neglected Tropical Diseases developing the process for the adoption of additional diseases as NTDs in 2016 (WHO, 2016a). The criteria largely repeat commonalities in the first WHO report (2010), adding further detail as Relman and Choffnes did above. However, the wording emphasises the poverty element about the disproportionate effect of NTDs on populations living in poverty to justify a global response (ibid.). A return is also made to the tropical and sub-tropical character in describing NTDs. Neglect by research is also still there, and the point is made stronger in saying that the research allocation is unfair, particularly in "new diagnostics, medicines and other control tools" (ibid.). Therefore, lack of options for intervention and advancements in existing technologies (e.g. diagnostics) is a problem, rather than there not having been groundbreaking research and viable control tools for many NTDs.

Some commonalities have notably been dropped, including the political voice of those affected, including the emphasis on stigma for girls and women, and the lack of NTD travel. This may signal the downplaying of a human rights element, while the major introduction has been the third criteria that the diseases "are immediately amenable to broad control, elimination or eradication by applying one or more of the five public health strategies adopted by the Department for Control of NTDs" (ibid.). However, this is under the proviso that relatively neglected by research is optional (i.e. 'and/or'). The mixed strategy for surveillance, control, elimination, and eradication of NTDs is acknowledged. What is left is neither solely a problem of research for new innovative solutions nor a problem of the attention, resource, funding, and implementation of existing tools. If neglect is both an outward signal and a symptom of neglect in research and implementation, what are the underlying causes looking at common definitions under themes and often presented in terms of the contradiction (e.g. between the poor and wealthy). See table 4.2 below:

Table 4.2 Definitions of neglect in the policy literature

a. Poverty and inequality: NTDs affect large numbers the poorest/marginalised, especially women and children but are not a problem for wealthy so do not receive the same attention as other diseases.	"NTDs are called 'neglected' because they generally are not considered public health problems in **wealthier** nations and historically have not received as much **attention** as other diseases" (NIH, https://niaid.nih. gov/topics/tropicaldiseases/, accessed 2/4/14).
	"*1* **billion people** are affected by one or more neglected tropical diseases (NTDs). They are named neglected because these diseases persist exclusively in the **poorest and the most marginalized communities**, and have been largely eliminated elsewhere and thus are often forgotten" (WHO, 2016a).
	"NTDs are a group of parasitic and bacterial diseases that cause substantial illness for more than *1* **billion** people globally. Affecting the world's **poorest** people, NTDs impair physical and cognitive development, contribute to **mother and child illness and death**, make it difficult to farm or **earn a living, and limit productivity** in the workplace. As a result, NTDs trap the poor in a cycle of poverty and disease" (CDC, https://cdc.gov/globalhealth/ntd/, accessed 2/4/14).

Table 4.2 Cont.

	"The people who are most affected by these diseases are often the **poorest populations**, living in remote, rural areas, urban slums, or conflict zones. Neglected tropical diseases persist under **conditions of poverty** and are concentrated almost exclusively in impoverished populations in the developing world. **Lacking a strong political voice**, people affected by these tropical diseases have a **low profile and status in** public health priorities" (WHO Features, https://who.int/ features/qa/58/en/ 012, accessed 2/4/14)
b. **Underdevelopment: NTDs have existed for a long time and reinforce poverty/underdevelopment through their impact/ cost.**	"These diseases, many of which have afflicted humanity for **millennia**, affect more than **1.4 billion people**. They **sicken, disable, and disfigure**, keeping people in cycles of **poverty** and costing developing economies **billions of dollars** every year. Until recently, NTDs saw little **attention** from all but a small handful of dedicated supporters" (Uniting to Combat NTDs, 2014). "NTDs are a diverse group of diseases with distinct characteristics that thrive mainly among the **poorest** populations. The 17 NTDs prioritised by WHO are endemic in **149 countries** and affect more than 1.4 billion people, **costing** developing economies billions of dollars" (WHO, 2013, accessed 2/4/14).
c. **Prioritise to solve: High-mortality diseases are given more attention, while NTDs disable/ debilitate rather than kill. Treatment cost is low through existing drugs, but new ones are also needed.**	CDC also present a 'Fast Facts' section on their website (CDC, https://cdc.gov/globalhealth/ntd/, accessed 2/4/14): 1 billion people across 149 countries/territories are affected (by at least one NTD) 100% of low-income countries are affected by at least **five simultaneously** 534,000 people are killed worldwide every year major disease burden, approx. 57 million **years life lost** to disability or death **treatment cost** for most NTD MDA estimated at less 50 cents per person, per year "Many neglected tropical diseases can be **prevented, eliminated, or even eradicated** with improved access to existing safe and cost-effective tools. Control relies on simple interventions that can be carried out by non-specialists" (WHO Features, https://who.int/ healthinfo/global_burden_disease/metrics_daly/en/, 2012, accessed 2/4/14) "NTDs are infectious diseases that generally are rare or absent in developed countries, but are often widespread in the developing world… The availability of **new safe and effective drugs** for NTDs could provide public health benefit for overall global health, but because these diseases are found primarily in developing countries, existing **incentives** have been insufficient to encourage development of new drug therapies" (FDA, 2014).

(Multiple sources, emphasis added)

Measuring for attention: from the 10/90 gap to DALYs

Many of the definitions of NTDs are related to poverty or underdevelopment and their lack of attention from governments, NGOs, and pharma companies. The solution is often also presented alongside the need for prioritisation, using existing safe and cost-effective 'tools', or developing new treatments. The lack of attention has been presented in terms of R&D for NTDs through the so-called '10/90 gap', which refers to resource allocation of global R&D compared with the disease burden.

The 10/90 gap is the finding of a report by 'The Global Forum for Health Research' in 2004, stating only 10% expenditure on global R&D is dedicated to problems that primarily affect the poorest 90% of the world's population. The 10/90 gap only reflects R&D, with the argument that the market share of pharmaceutical businesses is too small for the 90% of the world who are poor, as pharma lacks profit incentive (Liese et al., 2010). Smith calls the 10/90 gap "(A) staggering example of neglect … International aid couldn't just be the distribution of existing cures. It needed broad innovation" (2015). Here, it is a mismatch between needs and investment that mark NTDs out and so became a part of the argumentation that the problem of NTDs lies in R&D (Bosman & Mwinga, 2000; Hotez & Pecoul, 2010; Kilama, 2009; Unite for sight, n.d.). Even if the 10/90 gap is not explicitly mentioned, the unequal research spending by pharma is frequently referred to in media articles on NTDs (Balasegaram et al., 2008).

The 10/90 gap, as a measure, marked the beginning of metrics being used in relation to NTDs, to make a policy case for attention. R&D disparity is an important inclusion because it is in this context that neglect becomes striking, and a metric can be attached. On the other side, a lack of metrics for NTD burden was seen as a disadvantage. The WHO in 2007 stated: "Lack of reliable statistics on the burden of NTDs has hampered raising awareness of decision-makers on NTDs and zoonoses. Accurate assessment of the disease burden is crucial to prioritise use of limited resources, provide timely treatments and prevent diseases" (WHO, 2007, p. 14). However, it is more than simply representing reality.

The health economist, Christopher Murray, has been an influential figure behind the drive for better tools for measurement in health. The Gates Foundation invested in the Seattle-based Institute for Health Metrics and Evaluation where Murray is Director. In some part, NTDs have also been influential for Murray. In fact, Murray met Kenneth Warren, the director of the GND, in the mid-1980s. These were his thoughts on the programme:

> I think the GND program had a great effect. He coined the term and it has stuck, and now people compete to call their disease 'neglected'; there is a bit of a war about what the borders are, what is in and what is not.

Is leprosy neglected? Is rabies? There are a lot of different definitions of what is neglected, and I think that the concept can reasonably be traced back to Ken.

(Keating, 2014, p. S28)

Furthermore, the NTD schistosomiasis was somewhat of a catalyst for Murray in his journey to create the DALY metric, which stands for disability-adjusted life year. The DALY is described as a "... measurement of the gap between current health status and an ideal health situation where the entire population lives to an advanced age, free of disease and disability" (WHO Programmes, 2015b,). The part-biographical account *Epic Measures* (Smith, 2015) depicted how Murray had travelled with his family to South Africa and had been horrified after bringing a sick man to hospital, where his stomach had exploded – a severe complication of schistosomiasis. It stuck with him that the disease he had not even heard about before could be so devastating.

DALYs were developed by the World Bank and the WHO in 1993 through the *Global Disease Burden Study* led by Murray with Alan Lopez (ibid.). Murray describes that: "The original idea was you want a metric that can also be used in economic studies: if you spend X amount of money, this is how much health you'll get" (ibid.). Building on the earlier QALY (quality-adjusted life year), DALYs are a measure of the "health loss in populations against a normative standard" while QALYs tend to be used to "quantify health gains for interventions" (Mathers, Ezzati, & Lopez, 2007, p. 2). Some regard QALYs as a better measure of "subtle morbidities and long-term chronicity" (Zhou et al., 2010, Part A, p. 16) but Adams makes the observation that "... a crisis of *funding* produced the QALY in the Global North, but I would argue that it was the crisis of *data* that produced its counterpart, the DALY, in the Global South" (2016, p. 27). In determining which diseases to bring attention to, the DALY has been crucial, while the QALY says more about which interventions to take.

The intention has also been said assist health priority-setting otherwise influenced by politics and other pressures. It is through the DALY measure that NTDs could be exposed, through their estimated burden of disease. These estimates renewed interest in the underlying epidemiological parameters, as NTDs mainly cause morbidity rather than mortality. The assessment of the average disability incurred by a diseased individual is crucial for correctly compiling data to global burden estimates. The disability weights (DWs) are based on a non-expert or patient opinion but were developed through 'highly educated' focus groups (Zhou et al., 2010, Part B, p. 59).

DALYs form a way to support a particular description of the world and how to act upon it. Through the description supplied by the DALY, morbidity is put on par or to a raised position as mortality, working in favour of NTDs to emphasise the size of this problem (ibid., p. 3). Now NTDs can be described as: "… the fourth most devastating group of communicable diseases behind lower respiratory infections, HIV, and diarrheal diseases – ranking higher than either malaria or tuberculosis" (The Henry J. Kaiser Family Foundation, 2015). How NTDs are more debilitating and disabling than life-threatening is captured, and further constructed as a grouping. Standardised estimates for years of life lost due to disease, injury, and risk factors over time calculate one DALY as equal to the loss of one healthy life year, to the sum of Years of Life Lost (YLL) due to premature mortality in the population and Years Lost due to Disability (YLD) for people living with the health condition or its consequences (WHO Programmes, 2015b). NTDs tend to cause more of the 'Years Lost due to Disability' than 'Years of Life Lost' (Hotez et al., 2014).

Still, the DALY does also highlight how the NTD grouping is not completely coherent in the four DALY outliers in rabies, dengue, leishmaniasis, and African trypanosomiasis:

1   Rabies is preventable, with vaccination also an option post-exposure;
2   Dengue has less than a 1% fatality rate if detected early and proper medical care is given. Currently there is no known cure or treatment; and a vaccine (Dengvaxia) has been licensed, although it has been marred by controversy (Gubler & Halstead, 2019);
3   There are three types of leishmaniasis. Only one of these, visceral leishmaniasis (also known as kala-azar), is fatal if untreated; but all are treatable and curable;
4   Lastly, African trypanosomiasis (also known as HAT or sleeping sickness) is difficult to diagnose and treat but has been controlled on the African continent through surveillance. There are two forms of HAT, depending on the parasite involved. One accounts for over 98% of reported cases, causing a chronic infection for months or years without major signs or symptoms. When evident symptoms emerge, the patient can have advanced disease (WHO Factsheet No. 259, 2015). The other only represents 2% of cases but causes an acute infection that develops rapidly and invades the central nervous system (ibid.). The YLL may be due to the low survival rates if surveillance to prevent the disease transmission fails.

These four diseases are not strictly disabling unless repeated illness and recovery times are counted. Rabies is the disease that clearly does not fit this profile because it will almost always lead to death if a person is not vaccinated before infection or immediately post-infection before symptoms appear. The only documented exception has been through inducing coma, called the 'Milwaukee Protocol' (Aramburo et al., 2011).

The DALY has the capacity to measure the disabling and debilitating nature of NTDs as a lower-income country concern, but also has an impact through the Global Burden of Disease (GBD). In the early years, NTDs did not show up very highly and the NTD community was 'dismayed' by previous WHO estimates (1999–2004) which assigned DALYs equivalent to conditions of minor global health importance (Hotez et al., 2014, p. 2). The year 2002 was deemed particularly bad as no NTD appeared in the 20 leading DALYs and led to a full revision of burden estimates for 2005 (ibid.). Hotez and Musgrove, in 2009, made the argument that because NTDs are identified contributing to or an underlying cause rather than direct cause of deaths, they were overlooked – for example, schistosomiasis may lead to death by bladder cancer. They also argued that uncertainty about prevalence and incidence led to under-reporting of YLDs.

Later estimates calculated that the DALYs attributable to NTDs were equivalent to US$56 million; however, estimates dropped again in 2012 to only US$26.05 million (see Molyneux, 2014, p. 176), constituting only 1% of the total global disease burden. There are several reasons for such a discrepancy. The first is in the geographic spread and how this is measured, as NTD rates vary (by nearly 1,000-fold) across regions because of a concentration in the poorest countries. A second point is that disease burden associated with long-term morbidity is determined by DWs and "(T)here is considerable dispute of the DWs attributed to NTDs, and some case studies have seriously challenged both the DWs for different diseases, but also the numbers of people afflicted" (ibid., p. 5). Also, direct pathologies associated with NTDs are not included, such as for cancer and neurological conditions, and contribution to other heath issues have been ignored, such as mental illness.

At the other extreme, "… the higher DALY estimates for NTDs elevate the status of these diseases to a level at which they could be thought of as the fourth leg to a table built on HIV/AIDS, tuberculosis, and malaria" (Hotez et al., 2014, p. 2). Collectively, NTDs can be counted together. As Hotez et al. document, the 2010 measure attempted to resolve the earlier different estimate and also include more diseases, to provide a resulting figure of 48 million DALYs for NTDs, compared with tuberculosis (49 million), malaria (83 million), and HIV/AIDS (82 million), the latter accounting for two of the world's major diseases (ibid.).

It is important to remember that the DALY measurement is a 'calculus of credibility', in that evidence is placed by policy actors on a hierarchy. DALYs similarly do not sit in isolation in creating the Global Burden of Disease index, ranking diseases according to their DALY score. Therein comes the importance of measuring and creating metrics, to be able to list hierarchal and relational problems for policy that allow, on a managerial level, comparison and prioritisation of funding and resources. This is where much contention lies, as political process of democracy demands advocacy and different groups to petition on the interests, values, and causes they support and to adopt the measurement language through the DALY metric.

The Gates Foundation now uses the DALY on a wide basis to help determine priorities and evaluate potential projects. By quantifying years lost to poor health, disability, and earlier death, morbidity (not just mortality) allows for an economic valuing of human life. The measure tends not to be used in economic analysis of cost-benefit, but for cost-effectiveness (Smith, 2015, p. 145). Gates recounted the influence of the 1993 World Development Report with preliminary Global Burden of Disease findings: "... 'It was just a graph that had, you know, these twelve diseases that kill', said Gates. These included leishmaniasis, schistosomiasis, trachoma – the leading scourges, preventable at low cost, whose names he'd also never seen before" (ibid.).

DALYs are a tool for statistical categorisation within the wider instrument of estimating the global burden of health (Gales and Lascoumes, 2007). However, there is a difference between the type of tool described within the NTD community, referring to interventions and a metric such as a DALY. This also resonates with public policy instrumentation in the problems posed and chosen path to make policy 'material and operational', orientating relations between political society and civil society.

Even if NTDs do not reach the top of the Global Burden of Disease, DALYs have increased awareness. Measurement advocacy started with the 10/90 gap, an argument of neglect of R&D, especially from big pharma. However, the narrative was largely about the injustice of funding for health research and not matching needs. More persuasively, DALYs have taken into account the particular needs associated with NTDs through their disabling nature, which had previously been overlooked on priority lists. The quantification of disability was novel in global health, and so the interweaving of DALYs and NTDs has been more successful.

Already, the second WHO (2013) report on NTDs referenced the 10/90 gap and the DALY measurement. DALYs transformed NTDs into commensurable diseases to be measured alongside the big killers: HIV/AIDS, TB, and malaria, where "(T)he calculated economic rates of return suggest that investment in control/elimination of neglected diseases produces an economic rate of return of 15–30%, and is capable of delivery on a large scale" (WHO, 2005, p. 19).

Neglect in measurement

The selection and operation of metrics are not "... a matter of simple technical choices", but a mode of reasoning (Lascoumes & Le Gales, 2007, p. 8). Not only do the interests behind a metric or measurement instrument choice matter, but also the relationship between metric, public, and politics. Lascoumes and Le Gales argue that it is a particular representation and problematisation of the issue at stake in metric choices, which tend to produce inertia to challenge the status quo (ibid., p. 10). Their observations question what is not being represented or problematised through NTD metrics.

On one hand, the representation of attention for NTDs, the DALY measure, was negative at first – in the Berlin report, the measurement of NTD impact was in fact a reason for their neglect, because they "... do not score high from a disease burden perspective, and this lies at the crux for their neglect" (Canning in WHO, 2005). Canning argued that NTDs have been subject to the moral imperative of the 'rule of rescue'; that we should prioritise diseases that pose an imminent threat to life, where chronic and non-life-threatening conditions are overlooked. NTDs were faring poorly in DALYs for the period 1999–2005 (Hotez et al., 2014). However, as the metric has grown in complexity, more NTDs have been included, as well as more detailed reporting on their disabling effects (ibid.). Similarly, through the growing pervasiveness of the metric (Adams, 2016), country mortality and morbidity has popularised the idea of morbidity as a major concern; and it is measurable, so action can be taken.

On the other hand, the representation of the 10/90 gap concentrates on pharmaceutical R&D investment but does not explain the lack of attention for NTDs from other sources. Why have donor governments and NGOs not invested in R&D for NTDs? As Canning already alluded to, governments and NGOs have been more concerned with high-mortality diseases, and NTDs are less attractive in policy terms. Therefore, neglect by those actors has been due to other diseases being of higher priority on policy agendas, so that attention was directed at reducing the high-mortality rates of the Big Three. To be an attractive policy proposition, advocacy for NTDs needed to shift attention from mortality: "... high return on investment, based on very low costs with a strong contribution to human capital, should attract the ear of finance ministers as the 'quick wins' are investment rather than consumption goods" (WHO, 2005, p. 11). DALYs have since also been utilised by advocates and NGOs in a switch in opinion for NTDs. Below are the types of headlines employed.

The End Fund an NGO:

> When measured in disability-adjusted life years, the NTD burden is greater than that of malaria or tuberculosis, and ranks among the top four most devastating groups of communicable diseases, along with lower respiratory infections, HIV/AIDS, and diarrheal diseases.
>
> (The END Fund, n.d.)

Scientist advocates Hotez, Fenwick, Molyneux, and others:

> By some estimates, the neglected tropical diseases are second only to
> HIV/ AIDS as a cause of disease burden, resulting in approximately 57
> million DALYs annually.
>
> (Hotez et al., 2006)

Instead of being problematised by DALYs as low in importance by being
comparatively low mortality diseases, they are characterised as high in importance by being high-morbidity diseases. The section that follows now turns to
understanding neglect in solutions that are posed in order to tackle NTDs.

Finding neglect in solutions: '50 cents per person'

If neglect is understood in how the policy problem of NTDs is defined, this
is assisted through measurement of R&D investment with the 10/90 gap,
and of disease burden through DALYs. To understand neglect in solutions
and what interventions make the most difference is shown in the historical legacy of the underdevelopment of vaccines and drugs. Some existing
drugs are old, in need of improvement, or require continuing research in
case there is drug resistance. For example, successful drugs such as praziquantel, to treat the schistosomiasis parasite, may now be developing resistance. Certainly, penicillin to treat yaws is at risk of resistance, with concerns
also in the difficulty of refrigeration as well as training to administer in
developing country settings (Broadbent, 2011, p. 55). Other strategies for
addressing these diseases are available, either as alternatives or alongside a
drug-based strategy. Table 4.3 shows what strategies are recommended by
the WHO for each disease.

There are five NTDs[18] that are being addressed primarily through Mass
Drug Administration (MDA) of anthelminthics and antiparasitics, along
with antibiotics. According to the NGO ENVISION, MDA is the "... administration of drugs to entire populations, in order to control, prevent or eliminate common or widespread disease" (ENVISION, n.d.). MDA used to
control NTDs has been hailed as an effective policy intervention, which the
WHO describes as a 'preventive chemotherapy' to regularly and systematic-
ally administer medicines to populations who may either have an NTD or be
at risk (WHO, 2012).

It is a cheap form of treatment at 50 cents per person, according to the
CDC, as "... one of the best buys in public health – with a low cost of about
$0.10 to $0.50 per person/year and the benefit of helping prevent or treat
several different diseases" (CDC, 2010, p. 2). As Warren Lancaster, a senior
vice president at NGO 'The End Fund', has put it: "for the donor community
that's a very attractive proposition" (interview with author, Lancaster, 2014).
Similarly, Alan Fenwick describes MDA at 50 cents per person as "... the

Table 4.3 Strategies by disease

Drug-based strategies	Buruli ulcer, leprosy, yaws, leishmaniasis, mycetoma, chromoblastomycosis, and other deep mycoses	Antibiotics or antifungals and surgery
	Trachoma, lymphatic filariasis, onchocerciasis, schistosomiasis, soil-transmitted helminths	MDA of anthelminthics and antiparasitics, along with antibiotics
	Scabies and other ectoparasites	Antiparasitics, antibiotics, antiseptics
	Snakebite envenoming	Snake antivenom
Environmental-based strategies	Cysticercosis/taeniasis, rabies, echinococcosis, foodborne trematodiases	Food hygiene and veterinary public health measures or animal management
	Chagas, dengue/chikungunya	Vector control
	Human African trypanosomiasis	Surveillance through mobile screening teams of at-risk populations
	Dracunculiasis	Safe drinking water, surveillance, awareness among affected and at-risk populations

(Compiled from information on CDC: http://CDC.gov.org; DNDi https://dndi.org)

best buy for public health" (APPMG, 2009. p. 14), acting as a marketing tool to 'sell' an attractive solution. It proved to be a successful pitch for Fenwick, when the 50 cents per person metric caught the eye of Alan McCormick, a partner at global investment firm Legatum, following an interview Fenwick gave to the Financial Times in 2006:

> ... a phrase from an interesting article on philanthropy implanted itself in his mind: that such treatable ailments 'do not need innovation but simply modest funding and a little imagination in order to distribute drugs to those in need' ... He was inspired by the idea that it might be possible to change the lives of millions, to free them from the burden of devastating illness, for as little as 50 cents per person.
>
> (The Legatum Group, n.d.)

The result was the Legatum Foundation establishing The END Fund as an NGO to finance control initiatives, and supplementing and creating new programmes in a bid to control or eliminate the five most common NTDs. However, the '50 cents per person' proposition is not problem-free. There is some worry about drug resistance from continued usage at this scale (Barry, Simon, Mistry, & Hotez, 2013) and acceptance by local communities dependent on positive and experiences (Malaria Consortium, 2014).

Many NTDs are treatable through antibiotics or antifungals[19] but environmental strategies are crucial and are part of well-functioning health systems, (including information/education, clean water, sanitation, early detection/diagnosis/case management, surveillance, control of reservoir hosts, social mobilisation, and the strengthening of partnerships). For lymphatic filariasis, in addition to MDA, the WHO recommends use of common table salt or cooking salt fortified with diethylcarbamazine (DEC) for one year in endemic regions, alongside vector control. Some diseases are in fact better addressed with environmental-based strategies, replacing drug-based strategies or supplementing them. For example, safe drinking water through surveillance and awareness among affected and at-risk populations is the preferred strategy for dracunculiasis.

Still, preferred strategies are changeable and dependent on resources, disease spread, along with research developments. In the case of onchocerciasis, vector control had been successful in the past but was no longer considered feasible or cost-effective in the remaining African Programme for Onchocerciasis Control (APOC)[20] countries, which is why MDA is now favoured. Also, for the mosquito-spread diseases Chagas, dengue and chikungunya, vector control has been the main strategy because of a lack of vaccines, (so this strategy may change as vaccines are developed) but also, because clinical symptoms are often not present until the disease has advanced, such that drugs are less effective and have side effects. Food hygiene and veterinary public health measures or animal management (e.g. deworming of dogs, vaccination of pigs) are the best strategies for cysticercosis/taeniasis, rabies, echinococcosis, and foodborne trematodiases (although MDA may also be required in areas with high infection rates).

Comparing environment-based and drug-based strategies, a number of points are striking in highlighting the diversity of these diseases:

1   The diseases that require mainly a drug-based strategy is limited.
2   There is difficulty in developing vaccines/drugs for diseases with a mosquito vector. Vector control strategies work best today, but this may change, and the development of vaccines needs to be considered against the amount of resources needed.
3   Food- and animal-related illnesses are overlooked when considering NTDs in policy, as they require social/cultural change.
4   A number of diseases are near elimination or eradication, requiring a large amount of resources (rather than disease control).
5   Outlier diseases have limited strategies of control.

This chapter has demonstrated that problem and solution definitions that are drug-based have 'policy appeal'. Metrics identify the policy problem of NTDs through the 10/90 gap of R&D for new drugs not being directed at the diseases of the poor, and DALYs to pay attention to chronic diseases. The metric of 50 cents per person, presented by NGOs such as The Global Network Against Neglected Tropical Diseases and global commitments including the London Declaration meeting in 2012, also emphasise drugs as a central strategy and encourage involvement of big pharma.

However, returning to the 20 diseases and analysing what are the preferred individual strategies for control and elimination or eradication, the drug-dominant strategy unravels as they apply to just over half of the diseases, and outlier diseases have limited strategies for control. Furthermore, even though vector control strategies may be effective, the technical challenge of developing vaccines or drugs for diseases with a mosquito vector is high. A number of diseases have had mixed strategies (both drug and environmental), which have been yielding results. Included here are diseases that are near eradication as a result of vector control, community-level programmes, and health education alongside drugs (guinea worm and yaws). These diseases now require continued funding and resources, rather than new drugs or the implementation of existing drugs.

Drug dominance

Clearly, a drug-based solution, emphasised by the measurement and quantification of neglect, forms a large part of the rhetoric of the problem – as a lack of R&D for new drugs or the distributions of existing drugs – but it has limits. This preference is evident when we return to the very definition of what is a neglected disease. Returning to the definition of neglect for NTDs, the research funding argument assumes already that neglect is primarily pharmaceutical neglect. Neglect from pharma companies is in missing drugs and other treatment, prevention, or diagnostic tools; but, as Broadbent suggests, it may not be the best identification of the problem or solution:

> ... people have said, look, not enough research money is being spent on these diseases and that's what neglect is, and, you know, we should fix it by spending more research money on these diseases ... it assumes that the way you're going to get rid of these diseases is by developing more drugs ... saying okay, we've got to spend more research money on diseases; that's not a way of working out how to cure or treat neglected diseases; it's a way of working out how to do so and make a profit from doing so.
> (interview with author, Broadbent, 2014)

In defining neglect, the concentration is on funding and resources and the potential for solutions to come about through R&D and innovation. Broadbent identified a commercial angle to this, in how research money and a profitable product are needed, rather than, say, social and political change, or more intangible changes. He argues on similar grounds that other approaches can be taken, including a consideration of public health systems and initiatives. This is especially true if there are strategies and public health tools available, so it is not about starting from scratch or thinking that only solutions produced through research are viable:

> ... there are many other things you can do about diseases. There are public health initiatives. You can just arrange your society in a way that, you know, people receive better medical care ... it just struck me that many of the neglected diseases actually are preventable as they stand ... none of the actual neglected diseases that are normally listed as neglected diseases, count as being neglected in that sense which is quite strange ... they're all things that we could do something about if we just, you know, built some better roads or, you know, delivered refrigerated penicillin in the right places.
>
> (interview with author, Broadbent, 2014)

What Broadbent appears to mean, by saying that none of the neglected diseases count as being neglected, is from a pharmaceutical R&D perspective, because effective interventions are available for many NTDs. If pharmaceutical companies have been placed in the driving seat for a solution for NTDs, this further pushes for drug-based solutions:

> ... if you look at the sort of interest of pharmaceuticals in this topic, I mean, you know, it's easy to sort of bash pharmaceuticals but, you know, ultimately they are not going to look for ways to help with neglected disease as simpliciter.[21] They're going to look for ways that will also make them money ... in some cases that's going to help, but for many things it's just not clear to me that that's ... automatically the case.
>
> (interview with author, Broadbent, 2014)

Donations of existing drugs are a common way that a pharma company can help with NTDs, but committing to R&D may be a more onerous step and also may not be the best use of resources, as has been argued for vaccine development. Yaqub and Nightingale consider this issue in depth: "... vaccines are difficult to develop and can cost $600m–$1bn to bring to market" (2012, p. 1). The point they make is that investment does not guarantee success; some poorly funded programmes succeed, and some well-funded programmes fail, therefore vaccine development cannot only be thought of in terms of supply and demand where incentives are required (ibid.). More research funding towards NTDs may not yield the desired results, and there is an opportunity cost in not directing resources towards other strategies that have proved effective. The pursuit of such public health 'absolutes' as vaccines or eradication has to be viewed in the same context applied to public health problems more generally: cost-effectiveness, short-term and long-term goals, priority lists, and wider health agendas.

This point is acknowledged by the WHO and other public health actors. Margaret Chan, Director-General of the WHO, said when opening the London Declaration in 2012, that previously we may have relied too much on drug donation: "It is one solution … but it is not the only solution" (Michael Regnier, 2012b). Other participants repeatedly brought up the urgent need for clean water and sanitation in the communities at risk from NTDs; but for big pharma, they now see their responsibility as met, as Haruo Naito, the President and CEO of Eisai, said: "Supply of drugs will not be the bottle-neck" (ibid.). Still, it is in the characterisations of NTDs, through 'tropical' and 'neglected' as categories that also constrain what the potential solutions to NTDs looks like. They invite a technology-based solution, which over-emphasise drug-orientated approaches in drug donation and MDA.

How can neglect be made sense of through these accounts? The quandary of exploring the tropical category is of why NTDs persist when they have been more or less defeated in some parts of the world. There are known ways of controlling, eliminating, and even eradicating these diseases. As countries have developed, they have been incredibly successful at tackling NTDs, par-ticularly through environmental interventions (sanitation, safe water, health systems, and infrastructure). There has also been an expansion of scientific knowledge directed at certain diseases. Certainly, a lack of drugs does not provide a full reason for why NTDs are a problem.

Uneven technological progress is a concern held by Nelson (2011 [1977]) who, mainly looking at high-income countries, asks why social problems per-sist, despite high levels of technological advancement in other areas. This proposition could be taken to a global scale: why do NTDs persist in some places and not in others? This is not to say that countries were on an even basis in terms of burdens from tropical diseases, but some countries have been able to control or eliminate these diseases – high-income countries in both non-tropical and tropical regions. A key insight from Nelson is to not only rely on political reasons for disparity, but also science-based explanations for why scientific solutionism applied to social problems is not always the correct remedy. The first point to make is the resource requirements and technical complexity of some NTDs. Dealing with NTDs may be possible through an enormous amount of resources – for example, with sanitation, water, and hygiene systems – viewed to be part of a development solution. Countries such as Saudi Arabia have been able to invest heavily in expensive seawater desalination to prevent schistosomiasis (Hotez et al., 2012), but these sorts of interventions are not feasible in lower-income countries.

Technical solutions, which tend to be drug-based, have seen some successes, but some of the diseases have still eluded scientists, in part because of scien-tific complexity. Mosquito vectors (causing malaria and dengue) and tsetse fly (causing Chagas disease and HAT) prove to be difficult challenges. As Scoones points out, drawing on early work by ecologist John Ford, the diffi-culty may lie in how "… disease, ecology, human practices and wider processes of development are deeply intertwined, and that narrowly focused efforts to eliminate the vector or parasite are doomed to failure" (Scoones, 2014, p. 2). NTDs are seen both as a problem of poverty that is for development to solve and a problem of knowledge for science to solve. Still, neither science nor development can be end solutions in themselves. Demographic change and urbanisation have brought back dengue as a problem in some higher-income countries; and a vaccine for rabies, often viewed as an ultimate technological fix (Sarewitz & Nelson 2008), has not stopped deaths increasing in recent years (Bourhy et al., 2010).

Conclusion: otherness of neglect

There are many different shades to the neglect of NTDs; but also considerations of difficulty (in technical solution), complexity (in the types of diseases, their different pathogens, vectors, changing environments), importance (how high is mortality and morbidity, how many are affected), a time element (what could be an outbreak?), and ranking (one intervention over another, one disease over another, other problem topics, which can be most political).

The sense, then, in which neglect is attributed to the diseases is crucial in showing how the problems and solutions have been imagined in various ways. 'Neglect' has been chosen, by scientists and others involved in the advocacy for these diseases, as the most compelling characterisation. In exploring the categories of disease, the 'neglect' depiction fits well because the categories 'tropical' and 'neglect' come from the position of *otherness*. The political aspect of otherness is contained in who gets to define neglect. These diseases are located where the viewer is not, in the other tropical world of neglect. In considering who neglects whom, there is the impression of a stronger force over a weaker. Therefore, who does the caring and why it becomes crucial; the other needs to be cared for, the neglected people as "those less able to demand services" (Detels & Gulliford, 2015, p. 282).

The emphasis is on the lack of agency or power of the neglected. They are helpless and voiceless, as neglect in a holistic sense for a group of diseases does not lend itself to patient involvement. One party lacks care, where the pharma company fits this mould, as do the high-income governments and NGOs that are more interested in other problems. The perceived lack of care sometimes extends to the media and specific actors or structures, whether government officials or public health programmes.

Too much of NTD policy ignores endemic countries themselves. This is the next step in uncovering where neglect lies – questioning the role and understandings of disease are a reminder that NTDs affect poor communities to varying degrees and will be experienced as a problem alongside a host of other problems, some with greater priority than others. Certain values are engrained in the construction of NTDs in an assignment of blame and responsibility, invisibility and visibility, voiceless and empowerment, attention and inattention, and stigma and acceptance.

Therefore, the concept of neglect is problematic to use in universalist terms, as it is a subjective state affected by localised or national understandings. Should it then be left to individual countries to define neglect? Chapter 5 concentrates on the agency taken to address neglect through advocates and scientists within endemic countries.

Notes

1 Imperialism is the idea driving the practice, as Ake describes, it constitutes the, "... subordination of one country to another or at any rate the attempt to subordinate one country to another in order to maintain a relationship of unequal exchange. The subordination may be military, economic, political, cultural, or some combination of these" (1982, p. 136).
2 The treaty was signed at the end of the 'Seven Years' War', with Great Britain victorious over France and Spain, marking a new dominance of Britain and expanding to have a global empire (see Blackburn, 1988).
3 Manson developed the 'mosquito theory' of infectious disease transmission, founded the LSHTM in 1899, and was the first president of the Royal Society. Tropical diseases reflect partly the older tradition of 'diseases of warm climates', and Manson placed an emphasis on the European coping with a tropical environment than what came to be the colonial project of tropical medicine – a more all-encompassing programme of health and sanitation. However, while reflecting on the older tradition, Manson wanted to break with the medico-geographical distinction and bring in modern scientific grounds for differences in disease in temperate and tropical climates (see Edmond, 2006).
4 The sub-categories he outlined were fevers, general diseases of undetermined nature, abdominal diseases, infective granulomatous diseases, animal parasites and associated diseases, intestinal parasites, skin diseases, and local diseases of uncertain nature. One undetermined disease was the yet to be discovered cause of sleeping sickness (human African trypanosomiasis) transmitted by the tsetse fly.
5 In the latest edition of Manson's book in 2013 (Farrar et al., 2013), the sub-categories largely remain viral infections (HIV added), bacterial infections (tropical rickettsial infections responsible for many undiagnosed febrile illnesses included), fungal infections, mycobacterial infections (TB would not have been especially tropical in Manson's time), protozoan infections (malaria), helminthic infections (schistosomiasis), and ectoparasites (scabies). These include tropical diseases not judged to be neglected: the Big Three (HIV/AIDS/TB) and malaria, and those in the Millennium Development Goals: nutrition and maternal/child health. Other health concerns in the tropics that now arguably compete with NTDs are non-communicable diseases (NCDs) and environmental disorders.
6 Attributed to be.
7 References to international medicine are made, although this tends to be under the banner of international health, referring to health for developing countries. The University of Oxford has an MSc programme entitled 'International Health and Tropical Medicine', as do LSHTM ('Tropical Medicine & International Health').

There is a journal called 'Tropical Medicine & International Health', and also a 'European Congress on Tropical Medicine and International Health'. NTDs could be now said to sit within global public health, as the current conceptualisation of international health.

8 Note: the US did not have the more deadly malaria parasite (*Plasmodium falciparum*) that was found in Italy and is what health officials tend to be more concerned about, although there is an argument that *Plasmodium vivax* should not be regarded as relatively benign because of how debilitating and sometimes life-threating it can be.

9 As the main malaria treatment at the time.

10 The Italian malaria campaign proponents described it as being based on "rational scientific methods", but the religiosity of the campaign was marked (ibid., p. 56). The health clinic doctors were told to be "… apostles of health and hygiene", and open air clinics held at the end of public mass were set up so that people could be "… treated, medicated and evangelized" (ibid., pp. 58–9).

11 United Nations Statistics Division, http://unstats.un.org/unsd/methods/m49/m49regin.htm#developed, accessed 2/4/14.

12 "A zoonosis is any disease or infection that is naturally transmissible from vertebrate animals to humans" (WHO, 2015).

13 'Why Arboviruses Can Be Neglected Tropical Diseases', in a group of diseases dominated by "… helminths, protozoa, and many tropical bacterial species" (2008, p. 1).

14 Emerging infectious diseases are identified by the WHO to have arisen in the last 20 years and were previously unknown (as well as being incurable). They include HIV/AIDS, hepatitis C, Lyme disease, hantavirus (pulmonary syndrome), and SARS (severe acute respiratory syndrome) (WHO 'Emerging diseases' https://who.int/topics/emerging_diseases/en/, accessed 2/4/20).

15 Certainly dengue is a more commercial disease relative to other NTDs, which is why NGOs such as Policy Cures use the semi-commercial label (Moran et al., 2012).

16 Meaning frequency in a population of elements signalling infection such as antibodies in blood serum (Merriam Webster Dictionary).

17 The Argentinian soccer player Lionel Messi spoke out about Chagas disease after watching an Al Jazeera documentary on the issue (DNDi, 2013, accessed 2/4/14).

18 Trachoma, lymphatic filariasis, onchocerciasis, schistosomiasis, and soil-transmitted helminths.

19 Buruli ulcer, leprosy, yaws, and leishmaniasis.

20 This programme has closed as of December 2015.

21 Means simply or plainly but in philosophical terms tends to mean 'plainly, without qualification' (Philosophy Index).

References

Adams, V. 1998. *Doctors for Democracy: Health Professionals in the Nepal Revolution* (Vol. 6). Cambridge University Press.

Adams, V. 2016. *Metrics: What Counts in Global Health*. Duke University Press.

Ake, C. 1982. *Social Science as Imperialism: A Theory of Political Development*. Ibadan University Press.

Amaral, I. 2008. "The Emergence of Tropical Medicine in Portugal: The School of Tropical Medicine and the Colonial Hospital of Lisbon (1902–1935)." *Dynamis* 28: 301–28. http://cat.inist.fr/?aModele=afficheN&cpsidt=20752077.

Anderson, W. 1996. "Disease, Race and Empire." *Bulletin of the History of Medicine* 70 (1): 62–7. https://doi.org/10.1353/bhm.1996.0001.

APPMG. 2009. "The Neglected Tropical Diseases: A Challenge We Could Rise to – Will We?" *Report for the All-Party Parliamentary Group on Malaria and Neglected Tropical Diseases (APPMG).* https://who.int/neglected_diseases/diseases/NTD_Report_APPMG.pdf.

Aramburo, A., R. E. Willoughby, A. W. Bollen, C. A. Glaser, Charlotte J. H., Suzanne L. D., K. W. Martin, & A. Roy-Burman. 2011. "Failure of the Milwaukee Protocol in a Child with Rabies." *Clinical Infectious Diseases: An Official Publication of the Infectious Diseases Society of America* 53 (6): 572–74. https://doi.org/10.1093/cid/cir483.

Arnold, D. 1996. *Warm Climates and Western Medicine: The Emergence of Tropical Medicine, 1500–1900.* Rodopi. https://books.google.com/books?id= GacOed9-kvIC&pgis=1.

Balasegaram, M., S. Balasegaram, D. Malvy, & P. Millet. 2008. "Neglected Diseases in the News: A Content Analysis of Recent International Media Coverage Focussing on Leishmaniasis and Trypanosomiasis." *PLoS Neglected Tropical Diseases* 2 (5): e234. https://doi.org/10.1371/journal.pntd.0000234.

Barry, M., G. G. Simon, N. Mistry, & P. J. Hotez, 2013. "Global Trends in Neglected Tropical Disease Control and Elimination." *Medscape.* https://medscape.com/viewarticle/808013_3.

Bewell, A. 2003. *Romanticism and Colonial Disease.* JHU Press. https://books.google.com/books?hl=en&lr=&id=SNAJfFIs7kgC&pgis=1.

Blackburn, R. 1988. *The Overthrow of Colonial Slavery, 1776–1848.* Verso.

Blaut, J. M. 2012. *The Colonizer's Model of the World: Geographical Diffusionism and Eurocentric History.* Guilford Press. https://books.google.com/books?hl=en&lr=&id=PVWZdtoBXOYC&pgis=1.

Boseley, S. 2012. "Drug Companies Join Forces to Combat Deadliest Tropical Diseases." *The Guardian.* January 30, 2012. https://theguardian.com/global-development/2012/jan/30/drug-companies-join-tropical-diseases.

Bosman, M., & A. Mwinga. 2000. "Tropical Diseases and the 10/90 Gap." *The Lancet* 356 (Suppl): S63. https://doi.org/10.1016/S0140-6736(00)92049-X.

Bourhy, H., A. Dautry-Varsat, P. J. Hotez, J. Salomon, H. Bourhy, A. Perrot, J. M. Cavaillon, et al. 2010. "Rabies, Still Neglected after 125 Years of Vaccination." *PLoS Neglected Tropical Diseases* 4 (11): e839. https://doi.org/10.1371/journal.pntd.0000839.

Brito, A. C. D, & M. D. J. Semblano Bittencourt. 2018. "Chromoblastomycosis: An Etiological, Epidemiological, Clinical, Diagnostic, and Treatment Update." *Anais Brasileiros de Dermatologia* 93 (4): 495–506. https://doi.org/10.1590/abd1806-4841.20187321.

Broadbent, A. 2011. "Defining Neglected Disease." *BioSocieties* 6 (1): 51–70. https://doi.org/10.1057/biosoc.2010.41.

Brutto, O. H. D., & H. H. García. 2015. "Taenia Solium Cysticercosis – The Lessons of History." *Journal of the Neurological Sciences* 359 (1–2): 392–5. https://doi.org/10.1016/j.jns.2015.08.011.

Bynum, W. F., & R. Porter. 2013. *Companion Encyclopedia of the History of Medicine.* Routledge.

CDC. n.d. "Global Health – Neglected Tropical Diseases." Accessed September 14, 2015. https://cdc.gov/globalhealth/ntd/.

———. 2010. "CDC's Neglected Tropical Diseases Program." *CDC Global Health Factsheet.* https://cdc.gov/globalhealth/ntd/resources/ntd_factsheet.pdf.

Chakrabarti, P. 2013. *Medicine and Empire: 1600–1960.* Palgrave Macmillan. https://books.google.com/books?id=BFAdBQAAQBAJ&pgis=1.

———. 2017. *Bacteriology in British India: Laboratory Medicine and the Tropics. Rochester Studies in Medical History.* University of Rochester Press. https://books.google.fr/books/about/Bacteriology_in_British_India.html?id=zCqAAQAACAAJ&source=kp_book_description&redir_esc=y.

Conn, B. 2011. "Neglected Diseases, Emerging Infections, and America's Global Health Century." U.S Department of State: Diplomacy in Action. https://state.gov/e/stas/series/180126.htm#.

Conrad, P., & Barker, K. K. 2010. "The Social Construction of Illness: Key Insights and Policy Implications." *Journal of Health and Social Behavior* 51 (1_suppl): S67–S79.

D'Arcy, P. F. 1999. *Laboratory on the Nile: A History of the Wellcome Tropical Research Laboratories.* Taylor & Francis. https://books.google.fr/books/about/Laboratory_on_the_Nile.html?id=J35sAAAAMAAJ&source=kp_book_description&redir_esc=y.

Desowitz, R. S. 1991. *Tropical Diseases: From 50,000 BC to 2500 AD.* DIANE Publishing Company. https://books.google.com.ng/books/about/Tropical_Diseases.html?id=kPKfAQAACAAJ&pgis=1.

———. 1997. *Who Gave Pinta to the Santa Maria?: Torrid Diseases in a Temperate World.* Harcourt Brace. https://books.google.co.uk/books/about/Who_Gave_Pinta_to_the_Santa_Maria.html?id=DsjZAAAAMAAJ&pgis=1.

Detels, R., & M. Gulliford. 2015. *Oxford Textbook of Global Public Health.* Oxford University Press. https://books.google.com/books?id=_ehcBgAAQBAJ&pgis=1.

DNDi. 2013. "Lionel Messi, Football Player." https://dndi.org/diseases-projects/diseases/chagas/voices-for-chagas/1581-lionel-messi-chagas-disease.html.

———. 2015. "Diseases & Projects." https://dndi.org/diseases-projects/diseases.html.

Dobson, M. J. 2015. *Murderous Contagion: A Human History of Disease.* Quercus Publishing.

Doctors without borders. n.d. "Neglected Diseases and the 10/90 Gap." Accessed December 20, 2016. http://blogs.msf.org/en/staff/blogs/lauralee-in-lankien/neglected-diseases-and-the-1090-gap.

Eddleston, M., R. Davidson, A. Brent, & R. Wilkinson. 2008. *Oxford Handbook of Tropical Medicine.* OUP Oxford. https://books.google.co.uk/books/about/Oxford_Handbook_of_Tropical_Medicine.html? id=Gy6WPwAACAAJ&pgis=1.

Edmond, R. 2006. *Leprosy and Empire.* Cambridge University Press. https://doi.org/10.1017/CBO9780511497285.

ENVISION. n.d. "Mass Drug Administration." Accessed December 15, 2015. https://ntdenvision.org/technical_areas/mass_drug_administration.

FDA. 2014. "Neglected Tropical Diseases of the Developing World: Developing Drugs for Treatment or Prevention." Center for Drug Evaluation and Research

(CDER). https://fda.gov/downloads/drugs/guidancecomplianceregulatoryinformat
ion/guidances/ucm269221.pdf.

Fotaki, M. 2010. "Why Do Public Policies Fail So Often? Exploring Health Policy-
Making as an Imaginary and Symbolic Construction." *Organization* 17 (6): 703–20.
https://doi.org/10.1177/1350508410366321.

Gubler, D. J., & S. B. Halstead. 2019. "Is Dengvaxia a Useful Vaccine for Dengue
Endemic Areas?" *The BMJ.* https://doi.org/10.1136/bmj.l5710.

Guha-Sapir, D., & B. Schimmer. 2005. "Dengue Fever: New Paradigms for a Changing
Epidemiology." *Emerging Themes in Epidemiology* 2 (1): 1. https://doi.org/10.1186/
1742-7622-2-1.

Harding, S. 1993. *The "Racial" Economy of Science: Toward a Democratic Future.*
Indiana University Press. Retrieved from https://books.google.com/books?hl=en&l
r=&id=CmJWBaANlsEC&pgis=1

Hen, M. T. 1989. *Tropical Medicine for International Health.* Keisō Shobō. http://
catalog.hathitrust.org/Record/002237526.

Hotez, P. J. 2011. *The Neglected Tropical Diseases and the Neglected Infections
of Poverty: Overview of Their Common Features, Global Disease Burden and
Distribution, New Control Tools, and Prospects for Disease Elimination.* National
Academies Press. https://ncbi.nlm.nih.gov/books/NBK62521/.

Hotez, P. J., L. Savioli, A. Fenwick, P. J. Hotez, A. Fenwick, L. Savioli, D. H.
Molyneux, et al. 2012. "Neglected Tropical Diseases of the Middle East and North
Africa: Review of Their Prevalence, Distribution, and Opportunities for Control."
Edited by Serap Aksoy. *PLoS Neglected Tropical Diseases* 6 (2): e1475. https://doi.
org/10.1371/journal.pntd.0001475.

Hotez, P. J., M. Alvarado, M. -G. Basáñez, I. Bolliger, R. Bourne, M. Boussinesq,
S. J. Brooker, et al. 2014. "The Global Burden of Disease Study 2010: Interpretation
and Implications for the Neglected Tropical Diseases." *PLoS Neglected Tropical
Diseases* 8 (7): e2865. https://doi.org/10.1371/journal.pntd.0002865.

Hotez, P. J., D. H. Molyneux, Alan Fenwick, Eric Ottesen, Sonia Ehrlich
Sachs, & Jeffrey D. Sachs. 2006. "Incorporating a Rapid-Impact Package for
Neglected Tropical Diseases with Programs for HIV/AIDS, Tuberculosis, and
Malaria." *PLoS Medicine* 3 (5): e102. https://doi.org/10.1371/journal.pmed.
0030102.

Hotez, P. J., & B. Pecoul. 2010. "'Manifesto' for Advancing the Control and
Elimination of Neglected Tropical Diseases." *PLoS Neglected Tropical Diseases* 4
(5): e718. https://doi.org/10.1371/journal.pntd.0000718.

Kamat, V. R. 2013. *Silent Violence: Global Health, Malaria, and Child Survival in
Tanzania.* University of Arizona Press. https://books.google.com/books?id=6XxO
AQAAQBAJ&pgis=1.

Keating, C. 2014. "Ken Warren and the Rockefeller Foundation's Great Neglected
Diseases Network, 1978–1988: The Transformation of Tropical and Global
Medicine." *Molecular Medicine* 20 (Suppl 1): S24–S30. https://doi.org/10.2119/
molmed.2014.00221.

Kilama, W. L. 2009. "The 10/90 Gap in Sub-Saharan Africa: Resolving Inequities
in Health Research." *Acta Tropica* 112: S8–S15. https://doi.org/10.1016/
j.actatropica.2009.08.015.

Killheffer, R. 1997. "Dr. Robert Desowitz on the Transmission of Diseases from the New World to the Old." Breakthrough Medicine. 1997. https://astralgia.com/webportfolio/omnimoment/archives/chats/bm061897.html.

Kropf, S. P. 2011. "Tropical Medicine in Brazil." Wellcome Trust: History. 2011. https://issuu.com/wellcome-trust/docs/wellcome_history_47.

LaBeaud, A. D. 2008. "Why Arboviruses Can Be Neglected Tropical Diseases." PLoS Neglected Tropical Diseases 2 (6): e247. https://doi.org/10.1371/journal.pntd.0000247.

Lascoumes, Pierre, & P. L. Gales. 2007. "Understanding Public Policy through Its Instruments? From the Nature of Instruments to the Sociology of Public Policy Instrumentation." Governance 20 (1): 1–21. https://doi.org/10.1111/j.1468-0491.2007.00342.x.

Lemaine, G., R. Macleod, M. Mulkay, P. Weingart, & W. de Gruyter. 1976. Perspectives on the Emergence of Scientific Disciplines. Walter de Gruyter. https://books.google.co.uk/books/about/Perspectives_on_the_Emergence_of_Scienti.html?id=PfotstpTldoC&pgis=1.

Liese, B., M. Rosenberg, & A. Schratz. 2010. "Programmes, Partnerships, and Governance for Elimination and Control of Neglected Tropical Diseases." The Lancet 375 (9708): 67–76. https://doi.org/10.1016/S0140-6736(09)61749-9.

Loomba, A. 2005. Colonialism/Postcolonialism. Routledge.

LSHTM. 2014. "Social Sciences Shaping Health – Interactive Report." https://lshtm.ac.uk/newsevents/features/2014/social_sciences_shaping_health_interactive.pdf.

Malaria Consortium. 2014. "Project Brief: Community Dialogues for Prevention and Control of Neglected Tropical Diseases." https://malariaconsortium.org/resources/publications/344/community-dialogues-for-prevention-and-control-of-neglected-tropical-diseases.

Manson, P. 1898. Tropical Diseases: A Manual of the Diseases of Warm Climates. Cassell and Company, Limited (Electronic Resource London School of Hygiene and Tropical Medicine). https://archive.org/details/b21356038.

Mathers, C. D., M. Ezzati, & A. D. Lopez. 2007. "Measuring the Burden of Neglected Tropical Diseases: The Global Burden of Disease Framework." PLoS Neglected Tropical Diseases 1 (2): e114. https://doi.org/10.1371/journal.pntd.0000114.

McCarthy, J. S., D. J. Kemp, S. F. Walton, & B. J. Currie. 2004. "Scabies: More than Just an Irritation." Postgraduate Medical Journal. The Fellowship of Postgraduate Medicine. https://doi.org/10.1136/pgmj.2003.014563.

McNeil Jr., D. G. 2012. "For Intrigue, Malaria Drug Artemisinin Gets the Prize." The New York Times. https://nytimes.com/2012/01/17/health/for-intrigue-malaria-drug-artemisinin-gets-the-prize.html?_r=0.

Merriam Webster Dictionary. n.d. "Seroprevalence." https://merriam-webster.com/dictionary/seroprevalence.

Mohammadpour, M., M. Abrishami, A. Masoumi, H. Hashemi. 2016, Sep 19. "Trachoma: Past, Present and Future." Journal of Current Ophthalmology 28 (4): 165–9. doi: 10.1016/j.joco.2016.08.011. PMID: 27830198; PMCID: PMC5093790.

Molyneux, D. H. 2014. "Neglected Tropical Diseases: Now More than Just 'Other Diseases' – the Post-2015 Agenda." International Health 6 (3): 172–80. https://doi.org/10.1093/inthealth/ihu037.

Molyneux, D. H. 2008. "Combating the 'Other Diseases' of MDG 6: Changing the Paradigm to Achieve Equity and Poverty Reduction?" Transactions of the Royal

Society of Tropical Medicine and Hygiene 102 (6): 509–19. https://doi.org/10.1016/j.trstmh.2008.02.024.

Molyneux, D. H., P. J. Hotez, & A. Fenwick. 2005. "'Rapid-Impact Interventions': How a Policy of Integrated Control for Africa's Neglected Tropical Diseases Could Benefit the Poor." *PLoS Medicine* 2 (11): e336. https://doi.org/10.1371/journal.pmed.0020336.

Moran, M., J. Guzman, M. A. Burke, & A. L. de Francisco. 2006. "Drug R&D for Neglected Diseases by Public-Private Partnerships: Are Public Funds Appropriately Distributed?" *Monitoring Financial Flows for Health Research 2005: Behind the Global Numbers.* Edited by M.A. Burke and A. L. de Francisco. Global Forum for Health Research. https://georgeinstitute.org.au/publications/drug-rd-for-neglected-diseases-by-public-private-partnerships-are-public-funds.

Moran, M, J. Guzman, K. Henderson, R. Liyanage, L. Wu, E. Chin, N. Chapman, L. Abela-Oversteegen, D. Gouglas, & D. Kwong. 2012. "G-FINDER 2012: Neglected Disease Research and Development: A Five Year Review." *Policy Cures.*

Mulligan, K., J. Dixon, C.-L. Joanna Sinn, & S. J. Elliott. 2015. "Is Dengue a Disease of Poverty? A Systematic Review." *Pathogens and Global Health* 109 (1): 10–8. https://doi.org/10.1179/2047773214Y.0000000168.

Mulligan, K., S. J. Elliott, & Corinne J. Schuster-Wallace. 2012. "Global Public Health Policy Transfer and Dengue Fever in Putrajaya, Malaysia: A Critical Discourse Analysis." *Critical Public Health* 22 (4): 407–18. https://doi.org/10.1080/09581596.2012.659722.

Musgrove, P., & P. J. Hotez. 2009. "Turning Neglected Tropical Diseases into Forgotten Maladies." *Health Affairs* 28 (6): 1691–1706. https://doi.org/10.1377/hlthaff.28.6.1691.

NASA. 1972. "The Earth Seen from Apollo." PhotographerNASA/Apollo 17 Crew: Taken by Either Harrison Schmitt or Ron Evans. https://nasa.gov/images/content/115334main_image_feature_329_ys_full.jpg.

Neill, D. 2012. *Networks in Tropical Medicine: Internationalism, Colonialism, and the Rise of a Medical Specialty, 1890–1930.* Stanford University Press. https://books.google.com/books?id=-PbUd0ooQSMC&pgis=1.

Nelson, R. R. 2011. "The Moon and the Ghetto Revisited." *Science and Public Policy* 38 (9): 681–90. https://doi.org/10.1093/scipol/38.9.681.

NIH. n.d. "Neglected Tropical Diseases." National Institute of Allergy and Infectious Diseases (NIH). Accessed September 14, 2015. https://niaid.nih.gov/topics/tropicaldiseases/pages/default.aspx?wt.ac=bcNIAIDTopicsTropicalDiseases.

Nunes, J. 2013. *Security, Emancipation and the Politics of Health: A New Theoretical Perspective.* Routledge. https://books.google.com/books?id=YfohAQAAQBAJ&pgis=1.

Packard, R. M. 2007. *The Making of a Tropical Disease: A Short History of Malaria.* JHU Press. https://books.google.com/books?id=B_V1Xj6wH7IC& pgis=1.

Parker, M., T. Allen, & J. Hastings. 2008. "Resisting Control of Neglected Tropical Diseases: Dilemmas in the Mass Treatment of Schistosomiasis and Soil-Transmitted Helminths in North-West Uganda." *Journal of Biosocial Science.* Cambridge University Press. http://eprints.lse.ac.uk/30641/1/__Libfile_repository_Content_Allen%2CT_Resistingcontrolofneglectedtropicaldiseases_Resistingcontrolofneglectedtropicaldiseases%28LSERO%29.pdf.

Parker, R., & Marni S. 2010. *Routledge Handbook of Global Public Health*. Routledge. https://books.google.com/books?id=RIqsAgAAQBAJ&pgis=1.

Philosophy Index. n.d. "Philosophy Index." Accessed September 14, 2015. https://philosophy-index.com/terms/simpliciter.php.

Pittalwala, I. 2014. "Breakthrough in Managing Yellow Fever Disease." *UCR Today*. http://ucrtoday.ucr.edu/25861.

Raphael, D. 2006. "Social Determinants of Health: Present Status, Unanswered Questions, and Future Directions." *International Journal of Health Services* 36 (4): 651–77. https://doi.org/10.2190/3MW4-1EK3-DGRQ-2CRF.

Regnier, M. 2012a. "Neglected Tropical Diseases: Action on All Fronts." *Wellcome Trust Blog*. https://blog.wellcome.ac.uk/2012/01/31/neglected-tropical-diseases-action-on-all-fronts/.

———. 2012b. "Neglected Tropical Diseases: The London Declaration." *Wellcome Trust Blog*. https://blog.wellcome.ac.uk/2012/01/31/neglected-tropical-diseases-the-london-declaration/.

Relman, E., & D. Choffnes. 2011. The Causes and Impacts of Neglected Tropical and Zoonotic Diseases: Opportunities for Integrated Intervention Strategies: Workshop Summary|*The National Academies Press*|*The National Academies Press. Forum on Microbial Threats; Institute of Medicine*. https://nap.edu/catalog/13087/the-causes-and-impacts-of-neglected-tropical-and-zoonotic-diseases.

Ring, N. J. 2003. "Inventing the Tropical South: Race, Region, and the Colonial Model." *The Mississippi Quarterly*. https://thefreelibrary.com/Inventing+the+tropical+South%3A+race,+region,+and+the+colonial+model.-a0117257653.

Rosenberg, C. E., & J. L. Golden. 1992. *Framing Disease: Studies in Cultural History*. Rutgers University Press. https://books.google.com/books?hl=en&lr=&id=agi08bNtBwgC&pgis=1.

Sarewitz, D., & R. Nelson. 2008. "Three Rules for Technological Fixes." *Nature* 456 (7224): 871–72. https://doi.org/10.1038/456871a.

Scoones, I. 2014. "The Politics of Trypanosomiasis Control in Africa." https://opendocs.ids.ac.uk/opendocs/handle/20.500.12413/6700.

Smith, J. N. 2015. *Epic Measures: One Doctor. Seven Billion Patients*. https://books.google.ch/books/about/Epic_Measures.html?id=EvqEoAEACAAJ&pgis=1.

Snowden, Frank Martin. 2006. *The Conquest of Malaria*. Yale University Press.

Stepan, N. 2001. *Picturing Tropical Nature*. Reaktion Books. https://books.google.com/books?id=tW7dNwfwkPcC&pgis=1.

The END Fund. n.d. "NTD Overview." Accessed December 21, 2016. https://end.org/whatwedo/ntdoverview.

The Global Forum for Health Research. 2004. "The 10/90 Report on Health Research 2003–2004." https://cabdirect.org/abstracts/20043112798.html;jsessionid=84A7B2585EFA800D7ADFF2BDA8298458.

The Henry J. Kaiser Family Foundation. 2015. "The U.S. Government and Global Neglected Tropical Diseases." http://kff.org/global-health-policy/fact-sheet/the-u-s-government-and-global-neglected-tropical-diseases/.

The Legatum Group. n.d. "United Voices: The Story of the END Fund." Accessed December 21, 2016. https://legatum.com/philanthropy/investing-in-development/united-voices/.

Unite for sight. n.d. "The Importance of Global Health Research: Closing The 10/90 Gap." Accessed December 20, 2016. https://uniteforsight.org/global-impact-lab/global-health-research.

Uniting to Combat NTDs. 2014. "Delivering on Promises and Driving Progress: The Second Report on Uniting to Combat NTDs." http://unitingtocombatntds.org/sites/default/files/document/NTD_report_04102014_v4_singles.pdf.

Ward, Andrew. 2014. "Sanofi Hopes for Substantial Reward as Dengue Drug Unveiled." *Financial Times*. https://ft.com/intl/cms/s/0/4f4197e6-2793-11e4-ae44-00144feabdc0.html#axzz3y6P9PPhM.

WHO. n.d. "Yellow Fever." Fact Sheet. Accessed May 10, 2020. https://who.int/news-room/fact-sheets/detail/yellow-fever.

———. 2005. "Strategic and Technical Meeting on Intensified Control of Neglected Tropical Diseases: A Renewed Effort to Combat Entrenched Communicable Diseases of the Poor." *Report of an International Workshop Berlin, 18–20 April 2005*. http://apps.who.int/iris/bitstream/10665/69297/1/WHO_CDS_NTD_2006.1_eng.pdf.

———. 2007. "Global Plan to Combat Neglected Tropical Diseases 2008–2015." http://apps.who.int/iris/bitstream/10665/69708/1/WHO_CDS_NTD_2007.3_eng.pdf.

———. 2010. "First WHO Report on Neglected Tropical Diseases: Working to Overcome the Global Impact of Neglected Tropical Diseases." World Health Organization. https://who.int/neglected_diseases/2010report/en/.

———. 2012. "Guidelines for Assuring Safety of Preventive Chemotherapy (First Edition)." The United Republic of Tanzania Ministry of Health and Social Welfare: National Programme for Control of Neglected Tropical Diseases (NPCNTD) & Tanzania Food and DRUGS Authority (TFDA). https://who.int/neglected_diseases/TZ_Guidelines_Assuring_Safety_Preventive_Chemotherapy.pdf.

———. 2013a. "Sustaining the Drive to Overcome the Global Impact of Neglected Tropical Diseases: Second WHO Report on Neglected Tropical Diseases." World Health Organization. https://who.int/neglected_diseases/9789241564540/en/.

———. 2013b. "World Health Assembly Adopts Resolution on All 17 Neglected Tropical Diseases." World Health Organisation. https://who.int/neglected_diseases/WHA_66_seventh_day_resolution_adopted/en/.

———. 2015b. "Zoonoses." WHO.

———. 2016a. "Report of the WHO Strategic and Technical Advisory Group for Neglected Tropical Diseases." https://who.int/neglected_diseases/NTD_STAG_report_2015.pdf.

———. 2016b. "The 17 Neglected Tropical Diseases." World Health Organization. https://who.int/neglected_diseases/diseases/en/.

WHO Factsheet No. 259. 2015. "Trypanosomiasis, Human African (Sleeping Sickness)." World Health Organization. https://who.int/mediacentre/factsheets/fs259/en/.

WHO Features. 2012. "Why Are Some Tropical Diseases Called 'Neglected'?" WHO. World Health Organization. https://who.int/features/qa/58/en/.

WHO Programmes. 2015b. "Metrics: Disability-Adjusted Life Year (DALY)." World Health Organization. https://who.int/healthinfo/global_burden_disease/metrics_daly/en/.

Yaqub, O., & P. Nightingale. 2012. "Vaccine Innovation, Translational Research and the Management of Knowledge Accumulation." *Social Science & Medicine* 75 (12): 2143–50. https://doi.org/10.1016/j.socscimed.2012.07.023.

Zhou, X. -N., R. Berguist, R. Olveda, & J. Utzinger. 2010. *Important Helminth Infections in Southeast Asia: Diversity and Potential for Control and Elimination, Part 2*. Academic Press. https://books.google.com/books?id=MWOI7z7m1M8C&pgis=1.

Chapter 5

Advocacy for neglect

A new disease brand

This chapter explores the means taken by scientists to address neglect by creating a new disease brand. The use of methods from commercial branding and marketing has become increasingly popular in public health (Crawshaw, 2013), where diseases and health causes are connected with brands and patients, or publics are treated as consumers. Considering the branding of diseases, Richard Smith, editor of the *BMJ* until 2004, reflected on changing his thinking about brand importance in medical contexts. He said: "Like most doctors, until recently I thought of branding as poppycock, an extravagant and narcissistic way of wasting money. But it's slowly dawned on me that I was wrong" (Smith, 2014). He had changed his opinion because "(A) good brand will inspire and prompt action" (ibid.) by providing meaning and purpose through an exciting visual or verbal form, with a compelling narrative. Smith had been convinced that awareness was not enough and that only appeals to emotion would evoke action.

The idea of simplifying a disease problem, including presenting a solution in an easily digestible form, can be seen with NTDs. A phrase on the website of the advocacy NGO the 'Global Network for Neglected Tropical Diseases' says: "While the problem is huge, the solution to NTDs is simple" (Global Network, n.d.). This solution relates to the NTDs where there are cheap, effective drugs available to treat a population through mass drug administration (MDA).

A brand begins with a name. Take diseases named geographically such as Zika, after the Ugandan forest it was first identified or Ebola, named after a river in Zaire in 1976 (Hotez, 2016a). These places will continue to be known through diseases. People can also be implicated in connection to diseases – for example, on the patient side. A clear instance of this type of connection was seen with the early names for AIDS, with serious socio-political implications: gay-related immune deficiency or 4-H disease, referring to 'Haitians, homosexuals, hemophiliacs and heroin' (Donovan, 1995). Or it can be on the doctor side. A rare neurological defect was initially named Hallervorden-Spatz disease after the Nazi doctors Julius Hallervorden and Hugo Spatz, who first described it after researching the brains of exterminated children (NDTV, 2013). This led to families affected by the disease to urge a name change to neurodegeneration with brain iron accumulation (NBIA) (ibid.).

According to Ab Osterhaus, a virologist, acronyms are another solution because they keep names short (Kupferschmidt, 2015). However, people often forget what the letters stand for, and they can still cause problems, as the WHO found in 2003 when they coined SARS – also a name associated with Hong Kong, officially called Hong Kong SAR (for Special Administrative Region). These might appear to be unintended consequences of naming, but the WHO does take disease branding seriously. In 2015, they urged naming to prevent inaccuracies and stigmas through best practices for naming new human infectious diseases (WHO, 2015). Keiji Fukuda, the WHO's assistant director general for health security, argued the guidance was necessary because of the emergence of diseases that can create "unintended negative impacts by stigmatizing certain communities or economic sectors" (Gladstone, 2015). Following the guidance could minimise negative impact on "… trade, travel, tourism or animal welfare, and avoid causing offence to any cultural, social, national, regional, professional or ethnic groups" (Kupferschmidt, 2015). However, others such as Christian Drosten, a virologist at the University of Bonn, points to geographic names sometimes being justified. It was clear to him that MERS, for example, was associated with the Middle East: "Would it have been better if we had named it novel betacoronavirus clade C, type 1?", adding "You should not take political correctness so far that in the end no one is able to distinguish these diseases" (ibid.).

Naming diseases is therefore both important and contentious. Scientists working on tropical diseases saw one reason for the lack of attention from the global policy community as being the name and brand itself. The weakness of the brand had been considered a number of times, specifically by a small circle of scientists influential in the field of tropical medicine, but also the WHO. Their contention was that these diseases have "complex, hard-to-pronounce names", and there was also the unresolved question of which diseases constituted the grouping,[1] with those most common or treatable making it into the majority of lists (Relman & Choffnes, 2010, p. 17). The scientists decided that these diseases needed to become a marketable commodity within a competitive market for public health resource. Simon Croft, a Professor of Parasitology at LSHTM, reflects on labelling to build advocacy and action:

> Other than the label, the NTDs have little in common … The NTD label has had major success in raising the profile of this group of diseases over the past 15 years through a combination of advocacy and scientific and public health programs. This has ensured that NTDs are on the agenda of major international organizations, including the WHO, the UK's Department for International Development (DFID), and the Bill and Melinda Gates Foundation, all of which have dedicated NTD programs.

In addition, organizations dedicated to NTDs, for example the Drugs for Neglected Diseases Initiative (DNDi, Geneva), have been established.
(Croft, 2016, p. 1)

Similarly, the WHO recognised the importance of "advocacy to change this situation" (WHO, 2007, p. 24).[2] By the time the WHO published their Roadmap policy document for NTDs in 2010, the writers remarked how: "(T)he NTD brand has proved to be a useful form of shorthand for communication" (WHO, 2012). According to branding expert Dorie Clark (Nordrum, 2015), NTDs act as a "brilliant umbrella term" because "(I)t allows funders to feel like they are addressing something important that has been hidden for a long time". NTDs straightforwardly convey a message of moral urgency, justifying funding. A number of (similar) interpretations exist about how the NTD brand came about. One account comes from an interview by the Wellcome Trust with Peter Hotez, President of the Sabin Vaccine Institute:

The phrase was part of a drive to think about these diseases in a fresh light ... After the launch of the Millennium Development Goals in 2000, a lot of attention fell on HIV, tuberculosis and malaria. Goal 6 called for action on those three 'and other diseases' ... but those of us working on the 'other diseases' felt we were on the outside looking in. We were driven to think afresh, to 'rebrand' these conditions.
(Regnier, 2012a)

The main instigators have been named as those scientists who established the 'Global Network for Neglected Tropical Diseases' in 2005, including "Professor Peter Hotez, President of the Sabin Vaccine Institute, Professor David Molyneux, a lymphatic filariasis researcher at the Liverpool School of Tropical Medicine" (ibid.).[3] These creation stories documenting the emergence of the NTD brand point towards a small, concerted group of high-profile scientists who had been working on NTDs, usually specialising in one or two specific diseases throughout their careers, at top-ranking universities as well as at the WHO.

The stories of the origins of something new serves a purpose, either to reaffirm the perspective of those involved in the creation or to make a point about the object of creation. The 'scientist advocates' felt heavily involved in the creation of NTDs and because they had begun an agenda of high-profile advocacy and policy engagement. An initial profile in *USA Today* first put a spotlight on Hotez in 2009. This news coverage was followed by a Wellcome Trust blog article in 2012 (also including Molyneux and Fenwick) and then a number of similar interpretations about how the NTD brand came about, many in the popular press through news stories and articles in science magazines:

- 2009: 'This scientist's passion: Ending the scourge of parasitic diseases', *US Today* (Sternberg)
- 2012: 'Neglected tropical diseases: The campaign trail', *The Wellcome Trust Blog* (Regnier)
- 2014: "How Three Scientists 'Marketed' Neglected Tropical Diseases and Raised More Than $1 Billion", *International Business Times*, (Nordrum).

The 2014 news story also emphasises the three scientists as main protagonists (Hotez, Molyneux, and Fenwick). This is a business story in the International Business Times rather than a more specialist science publication. The focus is on the marketing and the amount of money raised (referring to the cost of treatments donated by pharma companies).

Creation stories also acknowledge the involvement of some actors and not others, depending on where the emphasis is placed. The role of the WHO in the creation of NTDs has not been emphasised. It is through their own publications that they highlight their involvement (see WHO, 2010). The key scientist from the WHO was Lorenzo Savioli, who was the director of the Department of Control of Neglected Tropical Diseases. Savioli, along with Antonio Montresor, and Albis Gabrielli wrote an article on 'Neglected tropical diseases: The development of a brand with no copyright. A shift from a disease-centered to a tool-centered strategic approach' (2011, p. 281). The authors pointed to Dr Lee, the newly appointed Director General of the WHO in 2003, as responsible for starting a process of paradigm shift in the control and elimination of NTDs. 'Paradigm shift' is the specific choice of words used to connote strategic involvement to change thinking (rather than adopting branding or marketing rhetoric in the direct words of creation or construction). Savioli et al. therefore describe this as a move away from a scientific classification of disease biology to a practical approach based on needs (ibid., p. 281).

It was central that the WHO was on board for such a change. After all, one of the key roles of the institution is to provide leadership on health, including categorising diseases into groups to base action. As Savioli et al. (2011) describe, it was a change in philosophical position about how diseases and their treatment were viewed, requiring reorganisation. Following the Berlin meeting in 2005, the 'Department of Control of Neglected Tropical Diseases' was established at the WHO. However, rebranding alone was not sufficient. How the diseases had been viewed and approached in the scientific community and the public was a change that began much earlier.

Careers in an unmodern or modern science

In comparison to what is now a growing public interest in NTDs, during the heyday of tropical medicine, public interest was at a high, including in the tropical medicine scientists themselves. Cook (2007) even goes on to call the focus on individual tropical medicine scientists a domination of 'prima donnas' and the press coverage of scientists was described by Worboys as extensive: "… mosquito-malaria work of Manson's disciple Ronald Ross had found the columns of the daily as well as the medical press" (Lemaine et al., 1976, p. 85). For the scientists during the colonial period, tropical medicine was often associated with a prestigious and exciting career. For the tropical medicine 'father', Patrick Manson, after first working as a doctor in a lunatic asylum, his way of seeking advancement was "… in the fashion of the age, through a career overseas" (ibid.).

This public attention and career prestige would be followed by a wavering of interest, post-empire, to reach a low point in the 1970s when the diseases were associated with 'unmodern science'. Tropical diseases only began to see a professional renaissance in the 1980s, a sea change engineered by several protagonists, one of whom was Kenneth Warren at the Rockefeller Institute's GND. The change in perceptions of a career in tropical medicine was noted by Warren's biographer, Conrad Keating, when interviewing Nick White, the Professor of Tropical Medicine at Mahidol Oxford Research Unit:

> … when he [Warren] went into tropical medicine in the 1970s as a doctor, it had a very, very low status, and today, certainly in Oxford and I think in London, the brightest and the best want to go into tropical medicine. Now, that is because of the application of science, the cutting edge of science … at the first meeting of the GND, so he [Kenneth Warren] got these people, young biologists, who'd never hear, didn't know anything about a snail or a vector, you know, they were just people who were in at this new science for some reason, and the two people he got to speak to them in New York were George Nelson, and another great giant of British parasitology, and they were able to infuse these people with incredible stories about, you know, being out in the field in South America, and getting these people sort of interested in tropical diseases.
>
> (interview with author, Keating, 2014)

In 1993, the doctor and science writer Robert Desowitz similarly spoke of the promises of a new molecular science with a mixture of loss and trepidation: "(E)xpertise has been lost; the last generation of truly experienced 'field hands' are leaving the scene, lost to age and disuse" (Desowitz, 1993, p. 16). The 'field hands' that he talks about spent their time in endemic countries and appeared to have a more direct link with the communities affected by the diseases. For example, the connection with hygiene and sanitation was more pronounced. As Worboys describes, in the early 20th century the European doctors had very different concerns: "(T)heir knowledge and practice was structured around clinical and hygiene concerns, not with advanced science and technology" (Bynum & Porter, 2013, p. 522).

Desowitz was wary of the new phase of scientific enquiry into tropical diseases, taking place both in the endemic and donor countries, speaking of a replacement: "… in the West and in the research centers of the tropics by the 'molecular types', more concerned with the exquisite intellectual changes of modish science than with seeking practical solutions" (Desowitz, 1993, p. 16). It is noteworthy how he related the new science with impracticality, as the change that new science brought was the loss of something tacit, borne through experience, compounded by the discontinuation of teaching of tropical medicine key competencies. Desowitz went on to question what biotechnology was promising and whether these promises were overly enthusiastic of the expected benefits.

His view strikes a chord with the sociology of expectations literature, where researchers observe that sociotechnical promises arise when a new scientific and technological field is emerging and there is a promise of "social desirability and warnings about its potential negation effects" (Lucivero, 2016, p. 37). Desowitz envisioned social desirability in the expectation of a 'quick fix', where:

> (T)he razzledazzle and promise of biotechnology have led Third World health officials to expect the quick fix – the malaria vaccine 'just around the corner,' the genetically altered mosquito that yesterday's press release proclaims will be the last word in controlling vector-borne diseases; and confusing diagnosis with cure, the DNA probe techniques to detect parasites even at clinically insignificant levels.
>
> (1991, p. 16)

To Desowitz, this promise was illusionary and produced negative effects in the distraction from more useful work: "(T)here is an imbalance, a discontinuity between research and reality. This is an imbalance that has inhibited improvement in the health of tropical peoples; but in addition, I believe it has actually contributed to the deterioration of health" (1991, pp. 16–7). These words were written is the 1990s when the transition from the practical 'field hand' to the 'modish' molecular biologist was just beginning within tropical medicine. The continued promise of biotechnology, in anticipation of a momentous payoff, is still in operation today (see Nightingale & Martin, 2004). Approximately three decades later, a malaria vaccine has inched closer, and genetically altered mosquitos have become a reality, although the eradication goal is viewed with a sceptical eye as time passes. There is less of a harking back to the old practice but a growing emphasis on basic science and the established techniques of testing on natural products.

The three 2015 Nobel Prize winners in Physiology or Medicine were William C. Campbell and Satoshi Ōmura, "for their discoveries concerning a novel therapy against infections caused by roundworm parasites", and Youyou Tu, "for her discoveries concerning a novel therapy against Malaria" (adapted from Nobel Prize, n.d.). Molyneux and Ward make this point when reflecting on the 2015 prize:

> No rational drug design was employed and no magic bullets were sought. No synthetic chemistry or targeted design was involved in the initial discovery of the active products. The current mantra from the community is focused on the need for new products emerging from our understanding of the science based on our 'omic' interrogation of these complex parasites and the identification of unique biochemical weak points for intervention. The fact that this approach has largely failed to date is not lost to most in the drug discovery area who can point to the success of ivermectin and artemisinin, drugs delivered through bio-prospection and ancient knowledge of herbal remedies.
>
> (Molyneux & Ward, 2015, p. 605)

Today, the recognition of tropical medicine once more, through the Nobel Prize winners, has been a boost to amplify the position of scientists; although it has also been a process of institution-building to raise the status of NTD scientists and where the origins of the NTD brand can also be found, in the Rockefeller Foundation initiative already touched upon in previous chapters.

Borrowing from the past: 'Great Neglected Diseases' – the proto brand

The NTD brand has now entered the mainstream, but also has a longer history. As Regnier points out, the first research paper to "use and define"[4] the term NTDs was published in 2005, and since then "… the phrase has become a standard part of global health vocabulary" (2012b). Before this paper, Hotez and others referred to a number of different terms including 'tropical infectious diseases' and 'parasitic diseases' (Hotez, 2002; Hotez et al., 2004). Why, then, was the concept of 'neglected' used for the NTD brand?

The wording, to some extent, was borrowed from the past; before NTDs were 'The Great Neglected Diseases of Mankind' (GNDs), running from 1977 to 2000. Coming from the Rockefeller Foundation, the foremost philanthropic organisation of that time, the GND name was compatible with the foundation's ambitious mission to promote the well-being of humanity. GNDs were making reference to the type of diseases that could be NTDs, including many parasitic diseases, as Hotez noted: "(T)he emphasis was on parasitic infections that plagued people living in poverty" (Keating, 2014, p. S32). The descriptions of these diseases are dramatic, to evoke emotion to situate these diseases on a global and historical level of importance.

In fact, the GNDs followed a similar definition to those commonly used for NTDs, as Kenneth Warren, the director of the GND, described: "These diseases are great in terms of the enormous numbers of people suffering from them and are neglected both financially and scientifically" (Warren, 1978, p 572). The emphasis is on the large numbers of people affected; but he also pondered on the type of neglect that was occurring – financial and scientific, how neglect was multi-causal, and that it is not only rare diseases that are neglected: "There are many reasons, other than rarity, why diseases might be neglected, which go far beyond the profit motive" (Kenneth Warren in Scheinberg, 1989, p. 169). This question still holds today – to the financial and scientific neglect identified by Warren, social and political could be added and are additional areas of neglect the rebranding has tried to address. Pharmaceutical companies and donors might be the obvious sources of financial neglect, and the interest of the scientific community the cause of scientific neglect. However, the media, public, and governments are also sources of neglect, socially and politically. For Warren, the financing was available to an extent with the Rockefeller endowment, so his emphasis was in garnering the attention of scientists and addressing the scientific neglect.

Furthermore, the GND was reflecting the changes in 'neglected' and 'non-neglected' tropical diseases. Malaria had already been downgraded during the lifespan of the programme to a "great 'relatively' neglected disease" (Warren, 1978, p. 176). Therefore, there had already begun to be a distinction between the Big Three and neglected 'other diseases'.[5] Keating believes that the origin of the word 'neglected' in the context of tropical diseases comes from the GND, which he admits is "… a rather grandiose title, but he invented really the lingua franca, so now, in your own case, this word 'neglected', this is where it comes from" (interview with author, Keating, 2014). This view is supported by others, including Simon Croft, who described how the concept of NTDs was first proposed by Warren to bring attention to "… a large proportion of the human population who were poor, who suffered from chronic, disabling but rarely fatal diseases, and who were often stigmatized and unemployed" (Croft, 2016, p. 1).

'Great' may also have been a more common term at the time to refer to disease. Norman Stoll (see Stoll, 1947) was a renowned parasitologist and epidemiologist based at the Rockefeller Institute who played a key role in bringing attention to the problem of parasitic worms in humans. He presented a paper to the American Society of Parasitologists, reacting to parasitic worm-infected servicemen returning from the pacific battlefields of World War II (Klass, 2015). He called these parasitic infections "the great infection of mankind" and highlighted the need to conquer worms for the common good and raise human capabilities: "(F)or only in a society made up of parasite-free individuals will we know of what the human being is capable" (quoted by Klass, 2015).

Indeed, both descriptions of the GND diseases are dramatic enough to evoke emotion in 'great' and 'neglected'. Even 'mankind' situates these diseases on a global and historical level of importance. For Keating, the man-kind encompassment that the GND made had a resounding effect on the dis-cipline, and it involved an inclusiveness of low- and middle-income countries to attempt to leave behind a colonial past:

> ... the whole idea of tropical medicine, to medicine and to tropics, has changed because of that [the GND], and I think if you look at the amount of papers that are GND produced, if you look at the amount of people who were funded in the developing world, it was about, of all the scientists in it, I think it was something like 56% were in the developed world and the rest in the developing world so it wasn't, this wasn't sort of colonialism, so in that way it was a much, much fairer system.
>
> (interview with author, Keating, 2014)

Later on, the phrase 'great neglected opportunities' was used by Jonas Salk, the US virologist who developed the polio vaccine (Warren & Bowers, 1982),[6] although not everyone was comfortable with the word 'great', which was viewed as grandiose but "it was great because the diseases were killing many people, children particularly, in the developing world" (Croft, 2016, p. 1). Similarly, Warren found that the GND term was not always well received in a marketing sense, as when he met with David Weatherall who was the founding director of the Weatherall Institute of Molecular Medicine[7] in Oxford in 1977: "... he didn't think it would ever really take off, and people, I think they were already thinking about neglected diseases ... from Weatherall's point of view it seemed an odd title" (interview with author, Keating, 2014).

Attracting scientific talent and the promise of biotechnology

The odd title did take off, but where the programme differed significantly from NTD activity today was in the core aspiration to bring in scientific talent, creating a network of high-quality investigators. The intention of the GND was to constitute a critical mass of talented scientists, attracting the brightest students, and conducting research of a quality that was rarely seen for tropical diseases in the 1970s (The Rockefeller Foundation, 1978). At the time, the view within in the community was that the most able and talented scientists were not directed towards diseases of the low- and middle-income countries. The call of the Rockefeller Institute in 1978 would aim to change this situation in asking for "... outstanding basic and clinical scientists to shift their attention to these great neglected diseases" (ibid., p. 25). Such an encour-agement of scientific interest on an individual level has appeared to have a lasting impact and may be why there is no longer the same need to actively attract scientific talent to NTDs.

Another aspect of bringing in the top scientists included applying bio-technology advances. Parasitology had once been at the forefront of medical knowledge but "... by the 1970s, the discipline had fallen behind the revolutionary changes ... in molecular and cell biology, genetics and immunology"; and Warren attempted to "apply modern biomedical technology in the understanding of the mechanisms of disease prevalent in developing countries" (Keating, 2014, S24–S25).

According to Conrad Keating, a medical historian and biographer, Warren stands out in the 20th century in associating 'modern science' with tropical diseases to challenge a "romantic, post-colonial attitude" to the new technologies, and molecular parasitology units were established among partners (ibid., S28).[8] Later on, Hotez would describe how the network went beyond setting up new units, to training new tropical medicine scientists and creating opportunities for collaboration. Keating argued that the ensuing tropical medicine collaboration happening on a 'global scale' had been unprecedented (interview with author, Keating, 2014). The GND formed a new geography of training in the next generation of tropical medicine scientists and in creating opportunities for collaboration:

> ... the activities of these molecular parasitology units would be integrated into a GND network that would meet regularly in Woods Hole or elsewhere. In addition to an extraordinary track record of scientific productivity and international scientific collaboration, the GND program and network trained an entire generation of scientists committed to tropical infections, many of whom remain close colleagues.
>
> (Hotez in Keating, 2014, p. S32)

Warren was making a parasitology network attractive through the meetings. Woods Hole, a US harbour town in Cape Cod, carried prestige but also acted as a retreat.[9] Hotez described the appeal of this network and the annual meeting:

> They had these fantastic annual meetings where everyone funded by the Foundation would come to Woods Hole. We would go to these meetings every year and I would get the chance to meet all of these extraordinary people. This meant a lot because today I am still in touch with a lot of these same people who have gone on to have distinguished careers in tropical medicine ...
>
> (quoted in Esch, 2007, p. 46)

See photo below of the GND members meeting in Woods Hole (in the early 1980s) (Figure 5.1).

Today, scientists researching NTDs know they will be applying cutting-edge science while also having the appeal of contributing to a social good.

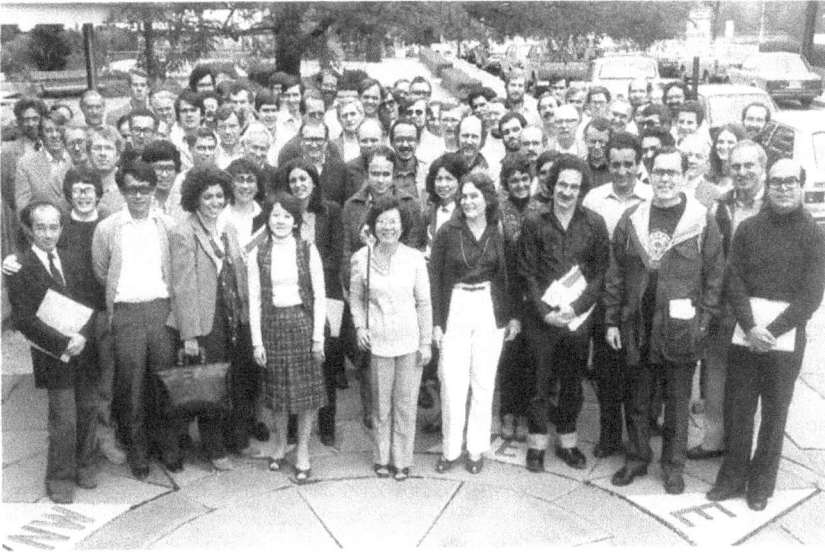

Figure 5.1 "A meeting of the Rockefeller Foundation GND program in Woods Hole during the early 1980s".

(Hotez, 2014, p. S32)

Furthermore, it is not only biomedical scientists who are attracted to the field but also statisticians, demographers, epidemiologists, and health economists who embody the application of 'new science' to form an important group, as the focus for NTD research has moved from scientific application to reorganising research and delivery structures.

As Warren describes, it would not only be the use of new techniques and application of cutting-edge science that would attract the new generation of scientists, but also invoking in them a "new spirit of humanitarianism" (Kreier, 2014, p. 337). Keating spoke of how ground-breaking the work of the GND was; but it was also an exclusive club of carefully selected scientists, so the chances to open the network or scale up the activity were limited and may have affected the programme's long-term sustainability. Still, the legacy of a small elite group of scientists has been impactful:

> ... one of the things that I think annoyed people about the GND was that it was a club. If you're inside the club it was this great feeling. If you're outside the club, you notice them. And I think there were accusations of these Johnny-come-latelys. People thought Warren was a kind of a Johnny-come-lately ... he was trying to magnify the contribution of the GND and some people would say, you know, that was politically

motivated but he certainly rubbed people up the wrong way. I think there was an element, and it's interesting, the quality of the cohort he chose have gone on to be people who have been enormously important in their separate fields ... I think that it was very influential that Warren himself has been neglected ... today, as we know ourselves, diseases are fighting to be put into this neglected square so he invented an interesting sort of language and he, himself, has been forgotten ...

(interview with author, Keating, 2014)

Warren had discovered, early on, the 'neglected square', as Keating puts it. He saw power in calling something 'neglected' to spur action. Warren's use of neglect is novel in that it brings to focus the advocacy of diseases to a much earlier stage. Instead of only saying something needs to be cared about, it is actively characterised as requiring that care. GND diseases bearing the label 'neglected' was the equivalent of a red flag to mark them out. It was not enough to present a problem and solution, but rather to characterise the state of the issue in the first place, in order to be concerned about problem and solution.

Even if Warren is now a forgotten figure, his influence is still being felt with the generation of scientists he sought to influence. One of them was Peter Hotez, a young doctoral student, now one of the leading scientist advocates behind NTDs. Hotez was inspired by a 1962 Rockefeller publication at the age of 14 which described hookworm as: "... 'The Great Infection of Mankind,' affecting 600 million people, he says. I thought, 'How can it be that this is one of the great scourges of humankind and nobody's working on it?' ..." (Sternberg, 2009). This view was further confirmed during Hotez's college years, with hookworm research being a 'great fit' with the GND programme (Hotez, 2014, p. S32). He was inspired by the work of the Rockefeller Foundation on GNDs, just as Warren had set out as an ambition with eminent young scientists of his day.

Therefore, the story of the branding of diseases is a longer one about directing research collaboration and the arrangements that allow research to happen. This research direction, to guide the progress of scientific enquiry towards public welfare for science, was not deemed possible by some (e.g. Michael Polanyi, 1962). However, Warren has shown the direction of science through the reorganisation of tropical medicine as a discipline and policy concern. Through his leadership in the Rockefeller Foundation, he had the remit and means to care about the GND diseases, identifying the problem and turning it into a scientific programme and network. The main gap he saw was the need to attract talented scientists who would apply advances in scientific understanding and technique. Warren created interest and encouraged biotechnology to be used by co-opting the next generation of scientists, which would form the roots of the next era of tropical medicine – but it would be the scientists themselves directing the action.

Two scientist advocates who have been instrumental in reordering the place of tropical diseases are the US scientist Peter Hotez and UK scientist Alan Fenwick. As discussed in Chapter 4, they originally 'coined' the NTD phrase, with the first use of the term in their 2005 paper (Molyneux, Hotez, & Fenwick, 2005). They sought to make others aware of the policy focus on Millennium Development Goals (MDGs) in 2000 to malaria, TB, and HIV/AIDS, and how other diseases were left out of the spotlight. This contrast led to the construction of NTDs as a worthy cause by scientists appealing to policy and an advocacy campaign to promote these diseases. The advocate role for scientists is addressed next.

United States: media-friendliness and scientific diplomacy

Hotez is part of the new breed of scientist advocate, although there have been historical precedents, and it is a continuation of a trend that has existed before. Individual scientists in the past have figure-headed campaigns and gone on to have policy impact, in a desire for their discoveries to be meaningfully recognised, and requiring engagement with policy and politicians, from Albert Sabin for the oral polio vaccine to Richard Doll for the connection between smoking and lung cancer. In fact, Hotez quotes Sabin at the beginning of his book on NTDs and is clearly inspired by his message: "(A) scientist who is also a human being cannot rest while knowledge which might reduce suffering rests on the shelf" (Hotez, 2013).

Scientists have also been deeply committed to causes such as climate change or anti-war advocacy in the 1960s and 1970s (Hart & Victor, 1993; Meyer, 1995). However, in these cases, they stand alongside many other interested voices. For NTDs, scientist advocates have not had this type of multi-stakeholder backing nor the same ownership over the policy debate. In previous cases mentioned by Sabin and Doll, their policy intervention is very defined and specified, as they did not consider a whole group of diseases but an intervention concerning one disease. Similarly, the figures of tropical disease in the past have also been limited in the individual policy points they tended to make for narrow influence.

Scientist advocates like Hotez are deeply engaged in policy, coining, and popularising concepts about NTDs in order to put into policy or journalistic terms the issues they care deeply about. Hotez is a prolific writer and commentator in the media.[10] To provide an idea of his scale of work, as of 2021, Hotez published over 30 articles about NTDs, a large number of which are in *PLOS Neglected Tropical Diseases* (where he is Editor-in-Chief), many in specialist health journals and three high-profile articles in journals *Science* and *The Lancet*. The breadth of his media publication is wide, including mass media venues (e.g. *Huffington Post*, 2014a; *New York Times,* 2012b) and examples of more unusual connections between NTDs and other topics including the South China Sea (2016b); 2014 World Cup (2014), Global Christianity (2014a), and 'The four horsemen of the apocalypse: plague, death, famine and war' (2012).

The varying definitions for NTDs mean Hotez can write about these diseases in terms of defence, foreign policy, diplomacy, security, equality, religion, conflict, economics ... the list goes on. Often, they have similar messages presented differently. For example, 'vaccine diplomacy', about scientific collaboration for and as a result of diplomatic relations, is a topic he did not invent but has written extensively about (e.g. Hotez, 2008). As a US citizen, he is particularly interested in the American context, playing on the intersection between global health and foreign policy, which has proved to be fruitful. He has been a US Science Envoy, where he focused on vaccine science diplomacy and joint vaccine development with countries in the Middle East and North Africa (Pathak, 2014). As a leading force in the US in galvanising support in political circles and other realms of influence (e.g. academic endorsement with economist Jeffrey Sachs and celebrity endorsement with Bollywood star Abhishek Bachchan), he has played a role in building institutions such as the advocacy NGO the Global Network for NTDs, establishing the first US tropical medicine school (The National School of Tropical Medicine) and has been director of the Sabin Vaccine Institute.

His interest in tropical medicine began at a young age and transitioned into the new science era of molecular biology (Regnier, 2012b). Hotez has spoken of this journey to advocate in terms of signposts that have already been touched upon, with the portrayal of tropical diseases in popular science (the bestselling book 'Microbe Hunters' by Kruif, 2002) and the connection to Rockefeller:

> Well, I've had a lifelong interest in Neglected Tropical Diseases although they were not originally called that. I've had interest in tropical diseases ever since I was in my adolescence, that's when I knew I wanted to study tropical diseases. I had read Microbe Hunters as a child and that had a big influence and by the time I was 13/14 years old I had a copy of 'Tropical Diseases' on my night table. So it's kind of an odd beginning ... and then went to the Rockefeller University and Cornell Medical College for their MBPhD program where I began to work on Hookworm infection.
>
> (interview with author, Hotez, 2014)

There has been a shaping of the tropical medicine discipline through these outlets: *Microbe Hunters* and Rockefeller University. The history of science book *Microbe Hunters* is also referenced by other scientists, including several Nobel Prize winners, as an influence in their decision to study medicine (de Kruif, 2002). Described as "... one of the most successful pop science books of all time" (Henig, 2002), it had a wide reach and was accessible for younger readers. The book venerated scientists as heroic adventurers and celebrated the momentous discoveries in tropical disease: sleeping sickness, malaria, and yellow fever. The author Paul de Kruif had been at the Rockefeller Institute. Similarly, Hotez had gone on to Rockefeller University,[11] although it was later that he would become an advocate for health. He described this change in the following statement:

> I've had a lifelong interest also in trying to develop vaccines for helminth infections [a subgroup of NTDs] and that actually began when I was MBPhD student. So, I very much started in tropical medicine as a laboratory investigator with no real intention of becoming a global health advocate; that actually happened much later in life.
>
> (interview with author, Hotez, 2014)

Hotez wanted to build momentum after embarking on a career in infectious disease and tropical medicine, and for him, the major part of advocating for tropical diseases was the renaming as NTDs: "The phrase was part of a drive to think about these diseases in a fresh light ... I think as scientists we are taught not to be advocates ... That's something I'm trying to correct" (Regnier, 2012). He described how this policy interest materialised to *USA Today*:

> One evening in 2004, in Geneva, Hotez found himself lamenting the lack of interest in parasites with Alan Fenwick of Imperial College London and David Molyneux of the Liverpool School of Tropical Medicine. Over dinner, they founded the Global Network for Neglected Tropical Diseases to yank these afflictions out of the shadows.
>
> (Sternberg, 2009)

While all had their areas of specialism within tropical medicine, they united under a common cause. Molyneux, Hotez, and Fenwick all focus on helminths, also known as parasitic worms, and have formed the biggest group of NTDs that received more airtime as a result, compared with the viruses (e.g. dengue), bacteria (e.g. leprosy), or protozoa (e.g. Chagas).

Other tropical disease scientists have laid the groundwork in the type of policy involvement with which these scientists have engaged. One of the big names was Donald Hopkins, former director of all health programmes at NGO The Carter Center. Sandy Cairncross of the London School of Hygiene and Tropical Medicine (LSHTM) gave this animated account of Hopkins:

> ... he got the idea and campaigned, and as an ex deputy director of the CDC he had enough contacts and influence to be successful. He and his colleagues would attend all relevant meetings of the World Health Assembly and lobbied all the country delegates to vote for eradicating guinea worm ... So they did a huge amount of advocacy and published

a large number of papers with titles such as 'guinea worm; an eradicable scourge'...

(interview with author, Cairncross, 2014)

Therefore, through the guinea worm (dracunculiasis) eradication campaign, the method of publishing in the popular press's attention-grabbing headlines already had some precedence for tropical disease. Advocacy went right up to former President Jimmy Carter who had become a strong supporter in eradicating guinea worm. He founded The Carter Center with wife Rosalynn, aiming to "advance human rights and alleviate human suffering", with guinea worm as their spearhead campaign (Hills, 2015).[12] However, Philip Coyne, a former World Bank medical expert who partnered with the guinea worm programme, notes the difficulty in how such an NTD was treated, even with the support brought by Carter:

... you know, back in the late '90s it was fairly obscure. I mean, you know, the CDC and The Carter Center laboured in almost total obscurity for years on this disease. And there were a lot of people that thought that it was a waste of time. It was a waste of resources to try and actually eradicate this disease ... Jimmy Carter brought in ... the influence and fundraising ability of The Carter Center and now we're this close [to eradication].

(interview with author, Philip Coyne, 2016)

The campaign reflects a culture of advocacy that requires high-level political influence. The lobbying environment of American politics may be why Hotez is a man on a crusade, through many high-profile connections from presidents to celebrities; and by 2008, he would have his own Presidential Initiative for Neglected Tropical Diseases established by President Bush and continued by President Obama (Hanson, 2008).

In the UK, the next example is of a scientist advocate, Alan Fenwick, who created an NGO as a means to intervene on the ground in endemic countries. The initiative comes out of an academic institution, so is an example of a university taking practical means, grounded in academic expertise, to address a societal challenge. This engagement is part of the wider social remit of universities (in the US, the predominance of private universities and trustees means there is arguably a less receptive grounding for this type of project).

United Kingdom: change on the ground

Alan Fenwick established the Schistosomiasis Control Initiative (SCI) at Imperial College, London. SCI is unusual as a public health intervention programme active in low- and middle-income countries because it was established by an academic and based at a university. Although, another NGO providing NTD funding information – 'Policy Cures' – was established by Mary Moran at the London School of Economics & Political Science, later transferred to the George Institute for International Health in Sydney, and is now an independent group.

For Fenwick, establishing SCI was putting his parasitology expertise into organisational practice. After working in Egypt for 15 years, helping to reduce the prevalence of schistosomiasis until it was no longer a public health issue, he wanted to apply this knowledge in other countries (Regnier, 2012a). However, he faced a roadblock in that schistosomiasis did not need further research but rather implementation that required the convincing of funders. As he put it: "Many organisations are interested in supporting research ... but this left schistosomiasis and others in limbo: most of the research had been done. We had the tools which, if implemented properly, could help some 200 million people in sub-Saharan Africa" (Regnier, 2012a). The emphasis on R&D was having a harmful effect in this instance. To relate this situation to another NTD, guinea worm, it has been noted previously that this disease is close to being eradicated without the need for drugs, vaccines, or other biomedical interventions (Barry, 2007).

Returning to schistosomiasis, new organisational arrangements were required through SCI. In 2002, Fenwick received funding from the Bill & Melinda Gates Foundation to buy and distribute praziquantel[13] (an effective schistosomiasis drug treatment) to endemic African countries (Regnier, 2012a). By introducing national control programmes, Fenwick wanted to test a proof of principle: "Will these countries implement control if given access to drugs and funding?" (Regnier, 2012b). SCI has proved to be successful in treating schistosomiasis and soil-transmitted helminths, leading to charity evaluator GiveWell ranking it as one of the top charities to donate to, mainly because of the 'cost-effectiveness' of the interventions and the need for funding.[14]

Regnier, from the Wellcome Trust, asked Fenwick in 2012 how he felt that it had been "... left largely to scientists to get programmes such as the SCI off the ground". His answer was: "I've never even thought about it ... It's invigorating. I passionately believe in treating schistosomiasis ... it will be impossible to achieve any of the Millennium Development Goals without tackling NTDs" (2012b). This feeling was similar for Hotez, with his focus on soil-transmitted helminths and vaccines. Both have had a prominent role to play in raising the profile of NTDs and have framed the approach to tackle NTDs.

Advocacy roles

When scientists enter the political arena, there may be resistance to the adoption of a role viewed to be outside of their remit, going against an image of neutrality and objectivity. There is also a perception that scientists do not want to take responsibility for social problems, but this is clearly not the case with NTDs. Some have viewed this type of advocacy as quasi-religious in character, with one interviewee describing Hotez and Fenwick as 'evangelicals' with a 'missionary spirit' (interview with author, scientist at LSHTM, 2014). This description not only conveys their commitment, but also the unfaltering single-mindedness of following a mission.

Undertones of religiosity are also why it can be claimed by some that NTD advocacy and interventions are undertaken with over-promise and optimism (Parker & Allen, 2011), without fully considering negative aspects of campaigns or non-technical causes of neglect. There is a moral basis for why NTDs may be pursued single-mindedly, and this is more than the charge of a lack of social science critique for NTDs. Keating also talked about "that religious thing" in considering the motivations of tropical disease scientists:

> These people are altruistic-minded. I mean, the idea of medicine is healing, you know, of healing people; but there are these things you see in the tropical group that maybe are not apparent as in another. You need that personal connection to care about somewhere far away from you that you don't get reminded of every day.
>
> (interview with author, Keating, 2014)

Religion and moral duty certainly have played an intermittent role in the motivations and vision for tropical diseases. In the early days of Rockefeller, scientists motivated by 'religious-moral impulses' were pivotal in the establishment of the Rockefeller Foundation and in driving the quest for a malaria cure (Desowitz, 1991, p. 171). With NTD scientist advocates, a religious rhetoric was not particularly present; but belief, commitment, and moral impulse were repeated themes:

> … after my medical studies, I did not follow a regular MD career. After ten years as Professor at the University of Brasilia, I went to Rio de Janeiro, invited as a researcher of the Oswaldo Cruz Foundation (Fiocruz), a 116-year-old institution affiliated to the Ministry of Health of Brazil. Fiocruz was created to fight endemic diseases that in the beginning of the 20th century were harming the economic development of the country. I wanted to do good science while at the same time addressing the needs of the poor.
>
> (interview with author, Carlos Morel, 2014)

> I was brought up into the 1960s when there was a tremendous amount of idealism to do something useful, I suppose.
>
> (interview with author, Simon Croft, 2014)

I just do what I think is right, I'm not on the bench doing basic science ... I see myself as an ideas person ... I think people publish things and nothing happens even though it's self-evident, so I feel quite strongly about this. I just do what I think is right and if people want to buy into it, that's fine.

(first interview with author, David Molyneux, 2016)

Even for those scientists not on the high-profile NTD circuit, many are called to advocacy. David Warrell, Professor of Tropical Medicine and Infectious Diseases at the University of Oxford, has been a leading figure in tropical medicine, who is not so much in the media spotlight and in policy circles, but answering the question of "What is your ambition in life?". After a well-established career, his response was, ultimately, to have an impact on disease burden: "To improve the treatment and prevention of forgotten and unfashionable diseases like snakebite and rabies. They have too few champions and sponsors" (Shakur, 2005).

While scientist advocates introduced a new disease brand, with an early basis for this brand being in the GND programme, it also paved the way for a type of scientist advocate, shown through a profile of Hotez and Fenwick. Other actors such as pharma company scientists, not typically associated with advocacy, have also been engaged in advocacy for NTDs.

One precursor to the advocacy role for NTDs can be seen in the pharma company scientists (including a CEO) who pushed for ivermectin to be developed for use in humans and then to be donated free and indefinitely in 1987. Ivermectin is a drug to treat river blindness (or onchocerciasis) and was the first NTD drug donation programme, opening the door for many others. Collins stresses the part that they played: "... pharmaceutical company employees were often vilified as the industry came under fire for its astronomical profit margins and the rising costs of pharmaceuticals, these employees, like many of us, saw themselves as moral agents working within an ethical framework" (2004, pp. 104–5). The ethical work of pharma companies also plays a part in the 2015 Nobel Prize in Physiology or Medicine awarded to William C. Campbell and Satoshi Ōmura, although the involvement of Merck has not been well publicised.

From 1957, Campbell was employed by the American pharmaceutical company Merck, at their Institute for Therapeutic Research, and later, from 1984 to 1990, as Senior Scientist and Director for Assay Research and Development. It was Ōmura's isolated and cultured strains of soil sample streptomyces (obtained near a Japanese golf course) that Campbell found a component effective against parasites in domestic and farm animals.[15] The collaboration between Campbell and Ōmura was part of a novel international public-private sector partnership in the 1970s between Antibiotics Research Group at Tokyo's Kitasato Institute and Merck, Sharp and Dohme (MSD) in the US (Crump & Ōmura, 2011).

Ivermectin[16] was developed by Merck in 1987 (marketed as Mectizan) (Gill, 2012) and had become a 'blockbuster drug'[17] to treat animals for helminth infections, within two years generating annual sales of over $1 billion, "… a status maintained for two decades" (Crump, 2014). Once potential was found for humans, the company embarked on a joint research programme with the WHO (Collins, 2004). Merck engaged in a number of partnerships for distribution, including enlisting the help of former US President, Jimmy Carter, to act as marketer to high-level officials in endemic countries (Saporta, 2012). Such activities targeting an NTD had been isolated until then. When Merck decided the drug would be produced for free and made available for patients as long as it was required, it was an almost unprecedented undertaking. They had first pursued pricing the drug commercially before seeing this would not work for poor patients, and had unsuccessfully tried national and international organisations (e.g. the WHO, the U.S. Agency for International Development, the U.S. Department of State, European and African governments, and private foundations) (Collins, 2004). Merck senior management, particularly CEO Roy Vagelos, had been supportive throughout, and the scientists involved suggested the possibility of drug donation (ibid.). Some point to Vagelos originally being a university researcher, although it is not uncommon for pharma researchers to have previously worked in academia, while others attribute the move to organisational values:

> Abandoning the drug was unattractive both in terms of health benefits denied to suffering people in Africa, and in terms of characteristics of Merck and its situation: its corporate culture, its already-existing donation programs, and also its image now that many knew of the existence of this breakthrough …
>
> (Coyne & Berk, 2001, pp. 10–1)

Therefore, the pushing of the scientists and how Merck envisioned itself through its corporate culture led to the "largest on-going medical donation program in history", treating more than 60 million people annually (Merck website). Also, lymphatic filariasis, another NTD, is now being treated by ivermectin. Today, the Merck donation success story is used as a case study in business schools to illustrate an 'ethical dilemma' for companies in developing or distributing a drug for the poor, at cost to the company, while wanting to demonstrate social responsibility.[18] The donation did not begin as a dedicated research project but, since then, other pharma companies have followed suit with their own drug donation programmes for NTDs. Many of these programmes, similarly, are offshoots from commercial drugs for another disease or after no commercially viable market has been found (Coyne & Berk, 2001).

Scientist advocates in China and Brazil

In addition to the scientist advocates in the UK and US, scientists in low- and middle-income countries have also engaged in policy. Using examples not typically presented for tropical medicine research, both Brazil and China had important discoveries in tropical diseases in the 20th century and have undergone institution building. Scientists working on NTDs in Brazil and China have faced different environments with their own challenges, concerns, and visions to tackle NTDs, driven by differing histories and sociocultural values. Initially it may appear that there lacks a prominent role of scientist advocates in lower-income countries; however, this is not a full picture, especially when taking into account disease research histories.

To fully address questions of technology, science, and national identity in Brazil and China would be a vast undertaking. The aims here are narrower, to reflect upon how NTD policy is positioned and the characterisation of endemic country responses. Adams, Gurney, and Pendlebury have highlighted the growth and impact of research from Brazil and other emerging economies: "This establishes a new geography for NTD research with much benefit to affected populations" (2012, p. 3). Today, NTDs form a significant research topic and base of knowledge for emergent economies "because of obvious economic and social relevance … with a substantial volume of NTD papers in its portfolio" (ibid., p. 5). Brazil and China show some NTDs are relevant to some countries and not to others. This universalist treatment is a danger in having one umbrella category for disease; and the next question to ask is whose 'universal' is it?

Chagas disease, for example, has been a major concern in Brazil and schistosomiasis in China. As Yang et al. note: "Although schistosomiasis is neglected at the global level, this problem is not the situation in China. Political will, coupled with financial, human, and technical resources, has successfully controlled schistosomiasis in most parts of the country" (2014, p. 884). On the other hand, Chagas is only endemic in Latin America. There is also the re-emergence of dengue in both countries. São Paulo used to be free of dengue, but in recent years, there have been many cases, even in the richest areas, therefore the disease profile in the country is changing.

Other diseases that affect the middle- and upper classes – who are more heavily located in urban areas down the eastern coastal side of the country, spanning from Beijing to Shanghai, as well as growing populations – mean that NTDs face competition with non-communicable diseases (NCDs) (see Hotez & Ehrenberg, 2010). Yang et al. argue: "(N)on-communicable diseases dominate the public health arena in China" (2014, p. 881). Here, neglect is sometimes characterised as a competition between the new diseases of the wealthy and the old diseases of the poor (Singh & Singh, 2008). The rapid changes in the country pose new health risks and obligations. NTDs become less frequent in urban areas, meaning some medical schools no longer teach tropical disease pathology. One scientist in Shanghai described how the doctors are concentrating on non-communicable diseases: "They concentrate on heart disease and diabetes" (interview with author, Senior Researcher at Institute for Parasitic Disease, 2013). Emerging economies such as Brazil and China face their own unique challenges in dealing with NTDs, not only from the perspective of the specific diseases that are most prevalent but also social and demographic changes. The next section looks more closely at the individual countries.

Collectivist science in China

In China, the aspiration for science to be a means to national salvation has been well documented (Cao, 2004; Wang, 2002), but the view of the scientist has been more conflictual – tied, for instance, to political allegiances. This view is related to how the scientist is positioned within the national consciousness and a radically changing political climate for science. The emphasis of science is on collective effort, and the perception of scientists is still connected with (a not particularly positive view of) elites. Consequently, scientists have not played as active a role in policy and politics as seen in the UK and US. Collectively, the National Science Institute in China conducts basic and applied research, with the Chinese Academy of Sciences the main source of institutional prestige and clout. Wu Yishan, a chief engineer at the Institute of Scientific and Technical Information of China in Beijing, suggests that

> ... the negative connotation of 'politics' in China, deriving from a 'politics first' movement during the communist Cultural Revolution that was used as an excuse for various abuses, might be to blame: it is not that scientists have nothing to contribute, but that politics itself is tainted.

> (ibid.)

An example of the tumultuous past for the treatment of scientists during the Cultural Revolution can be seen through scientist T'ang Fei-fan. In 1957 the isolation of elusive agent for the NTDs trachoma was discovered but as with artemisinin, the treatment for malaria, it had not been known outside of China. UK scientists had been simultaneously working to pinpoint this agent until an article by T'ang Fei-fan et al. (from Tong Ren Hospital in Beijing), in a Chinese medical journal explaining the discovery, was stumbled upon by scientists (at the Lister Institute) (Cox, 1996; Taylor, 2008). What followed was an expansion in research on trachoma; however, around the time of China's Cultural Revolution (1966–76), scientists were unpopular. In the lead-up, there had been infamous communist purges of 'disloyal' subjects in the 'Hundred Flowers' campaign of 1956 when citizens were invited to express their views of the communist regime (Lu, 1969). This period was followed by the 'Anti-Rightist' campaign in 1957 – a crackdown of those critical of the regime and ideology. There are differing accounts of T'ang's death in 1956, after 30 years of work in parasitology and only a year after isolating the trachoma virus. Either it was by suicide, after being labelled a 'rightist', or murder.[19]

In celebrating T'ang in an article, Cheng et al. (2011) recount how the renowned British scientist and sinologist, Joseph Needham, said of Tang in a 1979 letter to the then director of the National Vaccine & Serum Institute of China:

> Dr. Feifan Tang (F. F. Tang) was indeed 'a friend to man' as our old English eighteenth-century phrase has it; he loved the Chinese people and was a doughty fighter in the fundamental field of preventive medicine. With all friends here, I salute his memory and I am sure he will never be forgotten in China.

The authors also note how he may have been overlooked until more recently:

> His research might have been continued for greater achievements if he had not been appointed to study vaccines of measles and poliomyelitis. Even so, he was still being questioned and judged. In 1958, he gave up his life to protect his integrity and dignity. Until 23 years later when Dr. F. F. Tang was awarded the gold medal by the International Organization against Trachoma, his great contribution became [sic] to be treasured. In 1992, the Chinese government issued a postage stamp in his honor. A bronze statue of Dr. F. F. Tang stands in front of the National Vaccine & Serum Institute, Beijing. It is a great pity that the trachoma study was discontinued in China for a while. Today, when we are in the new era of innovation, the lessons from our predecessors should never be forgotten.
>
> (Cheng et al., 2011, p. 350)

The science-politics tensions were obvious during this period, but also the 1950s through to the 1960s had been a peak time for NTD research in China. Successes included public health control measures against hookworm through the Hookworm Commission, leprosy with a nationwide leprosy programme, and then schistosomiasis, in an unusual campaign that saw peasants using sticks to remove parasite-carrying worms from riverbanks (Cox, 1996).

It remained difficult to separate science and politics, and a prominent example of the blurring of science and politics goes back to the 1960s. artemisinin, which has become a key antimalarial, had been discovered and isolated in leaves of the herb Artemisia annua. Despite this momentous discovery, artemisinin was kept a secret from outside. The drug was part of a large-scale secret government Project 523: "involving over 500 scientists in ~60 different laboratories and institutes" (Miller & Su, 2011, p. 855). The project combined western and indigenous knowledge enquiry to "... research and develop new drugs the Western way, screen traditional medicine and folk remedies to search for a Chinese therapy, and find ways to prevent malaria infection in the first place" (Hao, 2011). The programme had been devised to treat soldiers in the Vietnam War at the request of the North Vietnamese leaders; so, due to military intentions, it was shrouded in secrecy and also because "during the tumult of the Cultural Revolution, publication in scientific journals was forbidden" (Miller & Su, 2011, p. 855). By 1977, the work of the group was published, albeit anonymously. Secrecy continued until the Chinese economic reforms of the early 1980s, with the WHO only giving artemisinin endorsement in 2000 and was still not widely available until as late as 2006 (ibid.).

These accounts do not paint communist China in the most favourable light at a time of secrecy and isolation. However, a 2005 BBC documentary, 'Malaria Defeating the Curse' (Horizon), provides a more even-handed portrayal where the political climate involving China, the US, and the WHO all contribute to why artemisinin was held back. The point is made that it is not an ordinary scientific project, because the research was driven by politics – to assist the Vietnam war effort and encouragement by Chairman Mao to explore traditional Chinese medicine, rather than relying exclusively on western science. The protagonist in the story is Professor Ying Li from the Chinese Academy of Sciences (Shanghai Institute of Materia Medica), who commented:

> The foreigners seemed to be snooping. They were so arrogant and contemptuous. They were astonished that we Chinese had managed to achieve this amazing breakthrough when they had spent so much time and effort on it and failed.
>
> ('Malaria Defeating the Curse' documentary, Horizon)

There may have been just reason for suspicion as the US military were on the WHO steering committee for anti-malarial drug development, as the military has had a long history in anti-malarial drug development (ibid.). On the part of the western scientists, the element of disbelief may have partly been grounded in the uncertainty of accurate information coming out of China, including previously exaggerated claims about eradicating schistosomiasis and curing malaria with acupuncture (ibid.). Still, NTDs were a priority and The National Institute of Parasitic Diseases was established in this heyday. Established in 1951, it is one of the few institutes in China dedicated to NTDs as part of the China's Center for

Disease Control and Prevention (CDC) network, the leading public health agency.

Another aspect of secrecy has been that individual scientists were not well recognised. In later years, more attention has been given to individual actors on the international stage. Attribution has recently gone to scientist Tu Youyou for the discovery of artemisinin.[20] Tu was head of the research group at the Institute of Chinese Materia Medica for Project 523[21] and part of a national project against malaria. She received international recognition after being awarded the Lasker Prize in 2011, a prestigious medical award, and was the first Chinese person to win the Nobel Prize in Physiology or Medicine in 2015. While not being well known within China, the Chinese newspaper Wen Wei Po remarking how she had nearly been completely forgotten until 2011. Even Youyou herself has remarked modestly, and with nationalist sentiment, on receiving the Lasker prize: "(I)t is scientists' responsibility to continue fighting for the healthcare of all humans … What I have done is what I should have done in return for the education provided by my country" (McKenna, 2011).

However, despite the publicity of recent years, it does appear that government interest in NTDs has fallen. The scientists see underfunding as a major inhibitor to their work: "we have good drugs but not money to introduce into the market … we should be supported by government or international governance" (interview with author, Research director at Institute for Parasitic Diseases, 2013). At the Institute, despite having invested in more than 20 drug products in last 20 years, few are used in the field, and the scientists are frustrated they are 'just sitting there' (interview with author, Senior Researcher at Institute for Parasitic Diseases, 2013). This is not to say China has not had more recent successes against NTDs. As Professor Xiao-Nong Zhou, a senior scientist at the Institute, notes: in China "NTDs are one of the most prevalent infectious diseases, with more than 100 pathogens recorded to infect humans", but this situation is changing: "(D)ue to great efforts by government leadership, professional guidance and community involvement, NTDs have declined significantly with the increase in economic development in China" (2013). An example was the elimination of lymphatic filariasis in China in 2007.

To summarise, the confrontation of NTDs in China has followed a specific path affected by a changing political environment, as well as economic transformation in the country. From secrecy during the time of Chairman Mao to scientific recognition, and new health challenges, China has faced the NTD problem within a context of multiple concerns and influences. The renaming and higher profile of NTDs has provided an opportunity to reflect on successes, but as the China example has shown, individual countries' priorities will persist over global health prioritisation. In Brazil, similarly distinct interweaving of approaches to NTDs reflect the country's historical circumstance, political events, and sociocultural understandings of disease – particularly defined here through nation-building as a former Portuguese colony forming a national identify after independence in 1822.

Nationalist sentiments in Brazil

Tropical medicine in Brazil has been deeply seated in nationalism, personified through the pioneering Brazilian doctors Oswaldo Cruz and Carlos Chagas. They were two giants of public health in Brazil and in pursuit of NTD control and elimination. Cruz had previously been director general of public health in Brazil, which saw him introduce three successful sanitation campaigns against yellow fever, followed by a smallpox vaccination campaign in 1904. He was recognised by the international scientific community in 1907, at the 14th International Congress on Hygiene and Demography in Berlin, with the gold medal in recognition of the sanitation of Rio de Janeiro. As Carlos Morel, Director of the Center for Technological Development in Health at Fiocruz, points out:

> ... by propagating the role that science should play in the development of Brazil, Oswaldo Cruz managed to conquer and receive support from the highest political level [President Rodrigues Alves]; being nominated Director of the Federal Department of Public Health, he could efficiently fight the diseases that were devastating Brazil's economy, particularly yellow fever and plague.
>
> (Morel, 1999, p. 4)

Cruz went on to be the founder and director of the Oswaldo Cruz Foundation (or Fiocruz), a still-prominent public health institution established in 1900 (Fiocruz, n.d.). He was able to attract collaboration from scientists of high-income countries who came to work in the institute (Morel, 1999, p. 4). Moreover, this collaboration has been a lasting connection; in the visiting fellow programme and 'high-level scientist' programme with visitors from the US, Germany, and other countries (interview with author, Morel, 2014).

Chagas took over the directorship of Fiocruz following Cruz's early death at 45. It was Chagas, with guidance from Cruz, who discovered the parasite that caused American trypanosomiasis, later named Chagas disease. Morel highlights the deep significance of the discovery for Brazil on the world stage:

> How could one of the major medical discoveries happen in a poor country in the tropics, be published on the first volume of a local institutional journal and yet receive worldwide recognition and be one of the

seeds of a whole school of thought and research which still today has such a profound influence in Latin American science?

(Morel, 1999)

The discovery is highlighted by Krof and Sà as a

... symbolically significant event that represented the scientific project that Oswaldo Cruz sought to establish at Instituto de Manguinhos[22] ... it was acclaimed as a symbol of Brazilian scientific capability.

(2009, p. 14)

However, Chagas disease was also a symbol of the poor and vulnerable in the country being left behind. Chagas spoke of the scourge of disease that would bear his name, in relation to large sections of the population being "unable to participate in the progressive evolution of the country", and the news reporting picked up on this theme with headlines such as "Brazil witnesses a step forward for mankind and a step backward in the brutal reality, which the authorities need to address without delay" (ibid.).[23]

Chagas has enjoyed hero status since – a 'mythification' connected to the "... status and significance that the discovery and study of new disease played in the institutionalization of Brazilian medicine and science" (ibid., p. 24). His status, however, was not without contention, with doubts about the authorship of the discovery that some thought should have been attributed to Cruz, as the one who conducted the experiment (the findings of the Brazilian Academy later disproved this) (ibid., p. 26). His critics further argued against him on ideological grounds, saying that his idea of a 'diseased country' was exaggerated and pessimistic and would discredit Brazil abroad (ibid). Some have even argued that critique of Chagas prevented him from receiving a Nobel Prize (Kropf & Sá. 2009).

The interplay between science and nationalist ideas has meant that political events have deeply impacted scientists at Fiocruz. During the military dictatorial regime (1964–85), the country was thrown into upheaval; and in 1970 came the so-called 'Massacre of Manguinhos', when "renowned researchers from the Institute lost their political rights and were forced into retirement" (ibid.). The instability intensified in the 1980s, as the Director of Brazil's Center for Global Health at Fiocruz, Paulo Buss, described how the intertwining between medicine and politics became more pronounced in finding a role in the fight for democracy:

Our slogan was that Health is Democracy and Democracy is Health ... We organised a lot of meetings, putting together postgraduate courses in public health, civil society organisations, and so on. We felt it was very important to agree a construct of health as a right.

(Pincock, 2011, p. 1738)

Many within Fiocruz see the inclusion of health as a right to be important. Today, Buss has continued an outlook that health must be closely connected to policy and politics:

> I think medicine and society, as well as doctors and politicians, do not have very precise boundaries. There is no precise boundary between my work as a doctor of public health and my work in the field of social policy. This is the field where we can transform the world.
>
> (ibid.)

Along these lines, Fiocruz has been at the forefront of efforts for dengue with the 'Eliminar a Dengue: Desafio Brasil', part of the international not-for-profit research effort 'Eliminate Dengue: Our Challenge',[24] led from Monash University, Melbourne, Australia (Fiocruz press release, 2012). The scientists I interviewed in Brazil often spoke reiterations of the phrase: "It's not just science, it's social", and the context for dealing with these diseases, which included a culture of inequality in references to Brazil being the last country to abolish slavery.

Fiocruz remains the pre-eminent scientific and public health institution for research in Brazil and, arguably, Latin America (Fiocruz, n.d.). The Cruz-Chagas period represents what is viewed as a golden age in Brazilian research and public health, followed by attempts to emulate it since. Cruz and Chagas wanted to rival western countries in scientific achievement, but also to apply science to the deep social problems of poverty and inequality. Later, scientists at Fiocruz became politically engaged as doctors who were pushing for democracy. Better health was a demand that the government should provide for citizens, and as medical scientists and doctors, they saw themselves well placed to advocate for change. As the China example also shows, scientists in Brazil have been active in their involvement with tropical diseases, despite a sometimes-turbulent political backdrop. A political role in pursuit of other priorities overtook that of advocating for NTDs. What both countries therefore represent is an autonomous course in dealing with NTDs that is quite separate from the brand created to repackage the diseases.

This chapter has traced the emergence of an NTD brand, the pivotal role of scientist advocates in the UK and US, and ended with how NTD scientists are perceived in the endemic countries Brazil and China. In China, ground-breaking research by scientists was underacknowledged because of a sensitive political environment, and it has only been more recently that recognition has been bestowed. In Brazil, the relationship between scientific recognition and praise has also been contradictory, being intertwined with nation-building and the need to project a modern, disease-free state. The possibility of scientists taking on a larger role was constrained by these circumstances but also hampered by the way that a policy movement for NTDs initiated in high-income countries became 'global'.

A global policy movement

It was not a grassroots but an elite policy action that led to the raised profile of NTDs, through the scientist advocates that created a new disease brand. According to Sheila Jasanoff:

> Not all societal adjustments rise to the level of protest movements nor arise from below, as in the formation of group resistance; to the contrary, many salient adjustments in actors' identities, with profound consequences for the day-to-day conduct of society, occur within elites.
>
> (2005, p. 29)

Adams also wrestles with the idea that "... medical professionals have, by politicising their medicine, managed to advocate service to the people while preserving their own positions of elites in a still highly stratified and unequal society ... with their status as bearers of modernity" (p. 224).

However, the stories of T'ang, Cruz, and Chagas also show scientists who were caught in political conflicts about the ways that NTD research was approached within their countries. Their stories provide context to relationship between research and policymaking taking place in lower-income countries. Political upheavals and sociocultural changes have presented difficulties for NTD research and policy in China and Brazil. These developments are not well captured in the global policy movement for NTDs, while the globalising policy towards NTDs still relies on an idea of higher- to lower-income-country knowledge flows and donor-recipient relationships. For scientists in the higher-income countries, as has been explored, neglect is apparent in policy by donor governments, NGOs, international organisations, and through the pharmaceutical system. It is clear, however, that the capabilities of China and Brazil are both different to other countries and to each other. While the 'neglected' aspect of NTDs is more apparent from the perspective of the donor, it is not so much of a clear-cut case from the other side.

Notes

1   Addressed by the WHO in 2016 when they produced criteria for selecting NTDs (WHO, 2016).
2   In a 2007 report, their indicators for performance measurement included the fourth strategic area of 'Evidence for advocacy', which included, 'Increased media coverage of NTD issues' and 'Societal awareness about NTDs' (WHO, 2007, p. 24).
3   Others listed were "Dr Lorenzo Savioli of the World Health Organization, Dr Jeff Sachs at the Earth Institute, Dr Kathy Spahn of Helen Keller International and Dr Jacob Kumaresan, then at the International Trachoma Initiative" (ibid.).
4   The WHO did make a reference earlier (Remme et al., 2002) but did not consistently use the term or define it.

5 This is one dimension that remains a concern today: what is the level of neglect (neglected or more neglected) and at what scale (global or other) is a disease being addressed?
6 At a 1981 meeting of donor agencies and scientists in the Rockefeller Foundation in New York.
7 He was director from 1989 to 2000 with the centre named after him upon his retirement.
8 Keating, spent time with Warren's 'supporters and detractors', including many of the GND members and his wife who was present at most of his meetings.
9 Woods Hole is a convening place for scientific meetings (Marton, Fensham, & Chaiklin, 1994).
10 The majority of articles are co-authored.
11 Originally Rockefeller Institute, until it became a university in 1965 (The Rockefeller University, https://rockefeller.edu/about/history, accessed 2/4/14).
12 Carter lobbied for guinea worm eradication after encountering an infected patient in Ghana while still President (https://cartercenter.org).
13 This goes against some accusations of the foundation that it is uninterested in implementation, although the framing as a 'proof of concept' project is likely to have helped (The Lancet, 2009).
14 Although this ranking has proved problematic, as SCI was somewhat ambiguously labelled in the group of 'Top Charities without capacity to use new donations effectively at this time' in November 2019 because SCI had not identifi ed opportunities to effectively absorb additional funding (GiveWell, n.d.).
15 And purify that bioactive agent.
16 The bioactive agent was called avermectin and was subsequently chemically modified to produce the more effective compound called ivermectin.
17 These are "… medicines that bring in more than \$1 billion in sales every year" (Lorenzetti, 2016).
18 See for example, https://andrews.edu/~tidwell/bsad560/Case-Merck.html, accessed 4/2/21.
19 More information can be found in the archives of the Carnegie Council, where a writer in 1983 describes the contents of 'China Daily", which was (at the time) the People's Republic of China's two-year-old English-language newspaper: 'Page five is the Culture page, which, in the rhetoric of the New China, includes Technology, Science, and Medicine. One issue tells a chilling story about Tang Feifan (the Western version of his name, 'F. F. Tang', is given in a picture caption), who attained international renown as the isolator of the virus that causes trachoma. The article ends: "In 1958 Tang was unjustly accused of being 'reactionary'. On September 30, he committed suicide. His only son, Tang Shengwen, now works in the institute where his father devoted his life to research" (Hazard, 2009).
20 Although also forgotten were contemporary artemisinin researchers, Yu Yagang and Zhong Yurong. Researchers at Beijing university call for the "roles of others need to be further studied and established" (Hao, 2011).
21 Some numbers are believed to be auspicious in Chinese tradition (0, 2, 3, 5, 6, 7, 8, 9) – the same reason why the National High Technology Development Program contained these numbers.

22 The site of Fiocruz is on an old farm of 'Manguinhos'.
23 Held at the Academia Nacional de Medicina, electric lighting was used for the first time, "…a symbol of the Belle Époque prevailing in the recently refurbished capital" and disturbing footage of mostly children with neurological disorders, and the 'barbeiro' bug culprits to present an, "… antithesis of 'civilization' – in the center of medicine and capital of the country", with microscopes to see the new parasite (ibid., p. 25).
24 The project uses *Wolbachia,* a natural bacterium, introduced into the dengue-carrying *Aedes aegypti* mosquito to stop the virus from growing (ibid.).

References

Adams, J., K. A. Gurney, & D. Pendlebury. 2012. "Global Research Report: Neglected Tropical Diseases." *Evidence, Thomson Reuters.*

Barry, M. 2007. "The Tail End of Guinea Worm—Global Eradication without a Drug or a Vaccine." *NEJM.* https://nejm.org/doi/full/10.1056/NEJMp078089.

Bynum, W. F., & Roy P. 2013. *Companion Encyclopedia of the History of Medicine.* Routledge.

Cao, C. 2004. *China's Scientific Elite.* RoutledgeCurzon. https://books.google.co.uk/books/about/China_s_Scientific_Elite.html?id=uXA0mAEACAAJ& pgis=1.

Cheng, G., M. Li, & G. F. Gao. 2011. "'A Friend to Man,' Dr. Feifan Tang: A Story of Causative Agent of Trachoma, from 'Tang's Virus' to Chlamydia Trachomatis, to 'Phylum Chlamydiae.'" *Protein & Cell* 2 (5): 349–50. https://doi.org/10.1007/s13238-011-1050-1.

Collins, K. 2004. "Profitable Gifts: A History of the Merck Mectizan Donation Program and Its Implications for International Health." *Perspectives in Biology and Medicine* 47 (1): 100–9. https://ncbi.nlm.nih.gov/pubmed/15061171.

Cook, G. 2007. *Tropical Medicine: An Illustrated History of The Pioneers.* Academic Press. Retrieved from https://books.google.co.uk/books/about/Tropical_Medicine.html?id=iB_ibIXxhOMC&pgis=1.

Cox, F. E. G. (ed.). 1996. *The Wellcome Trust Illustrated History of Tropical Diseases. The Wellcome Trust: London.* Vol. 41. Cambridge University Press. https://doi.org/10.1017/S0025727300063110.

Coyne, P. E., & D. W. Berk. 2001. "The Mectizan ® (Ivermectin) Donation Program for River Blindness as a Paradigm for Pharmaceutical Industry Donation Programs." Washington: World Bank, World Bank Document - S17517en.Pdf. 2001. http://apps.who.int/medicinedocs/documents/s17517en/s17517en.pdf.

Crawshaw, P. 2013. "Public Health Policy and the Behavioural Turn: The Case of Social Marketing." *Critical Social Policy* 33 (4): 616–37. https://doi.org/10.1177/0261018313483489.

Croft, S. L. 2016. "Neglected Tropical Diseases in the Genomics Era: Re-Evaluating the Impact of New Drugs and Mass Drug Administration." *Genome Biology* 17 (1): 46. https://doi.org/10.1186/s13059-016-0916-1.

Crump, A. 2014. "'Wonder' Drug Attracts Global Health Award." *The Lancet Global Health Blog.* http://globalhealth.thelancet.com/2014/03/26/wonder-drug-attracts-global-health-award.

Crump, A., & S. Ōmura. 2011. "Ivermectin, 'Wonder Drug' from Japan: The Human Use Perspective." *Proceedings of the Japan Academy. Series B, Physical and Biological Sciences* 87 (2): 13–28. https://pubmedcentral.nih.gov/articlerender.fcgi ?artid=3043740&tool=pmcentrez&rendertype=abstract.

Desowitz, R. S. 1991. *Tropical Diseases: From 50,000 BC to 2500 AD.* DIANE Publishing Company. Retrieved from https://books.google.com.ng/books/about/ Tropical_Diseases.html?id=kPKfAQAACAAJ&pgis=1.

Desowitz, R. S. 1993. *The Malaria Capers: More Tales of Parasites and People, Research and Reality.* W. W. Norton. https://books.google.co.uk/books/about/The_ Malaria_Capers.html?id=Pr5sHdTh1JYC&pgis=1.

Donovan, R. 1995. "The Plaguing of a Faggot, the Leperising of a Whore: Criminally Cultured Aids Bodies, and 'Carrier' Laws." *Journal of Australian Studies* 19 (43): 110–24. https://doi.org/10.1080/14443059509387203.

Esch, G. W. 2007. *Parasites and Infectious Disease: Discovery by Serendipity, and Otherwise.* Cambridge University Press.

Fiocruz. n.d. "Fundação Oswaldo Cruz (Fiocruz)." Accessed August 13, 2015. http:// portal.fiocruz.br/en/content/home-ingl%25C3%25AAs.

Fiocruz Press Release. 2012. "Eliminate Dengue Partnership Announced with FIOCRUZ, Brazil." *Eliminate Dengue.* September 23, 2012. https://eliminatedengue. com/progress/index/article/195/type/media.

Gill, R. 2012. "A Call to Arms against Neglected Tropical Diseases (NTDs): The WHO Roadmap and Why Biotech Companies Should Invest in NTD R&D." *BiotechBlog.* https://biotechblog.com/2012/05/23/a-call-to-arms-against-neglected-tropical-diseases-ntds-the-who-roadmap-and-why-biotech-companies-should-invest-in-ntd-rd/.

GiveWell. n.d. "About GiveWell." Accessed November 10, 2015. https://givewell.org/ about.

Gladstone, R. 2015. "W.H.O. Urges More Care in Naming Diseases—The New York Times." *The New York Times.* https://nytimes.com/2015/05/09/health/who-reaching-for-political-correctness-in-new-disease-names.html.

Global Network. n.d. "Global Network." Accessed September 14, 2015. https:// globalnetwork.org/.

Hanson, C. 2008. "Presidential Initiative for Neglected Tropical Diseases." https://rti. org/files/fellowseminar/fellowseminar_ntdcontrol_hanson.pdf.

Hao, C. 2011. "Lasker Award Rekindles Debate Over Artemisinin's Discovery." *Science.* http://news.sciencemag.org/asia/2011/09/lasker-award-rekindles-debate-over-artemisinins-discovery.

Hart, D. M., & D. G. Victor. 1993. "Scientific Elites and the Making of US Policy for Climate Change Research, 1957–74." *Social Studies of Science* 23 (4): 643–80. https://doi.org/10.1177/030631293023004002.

Hazard, P. D. 2009. "The 'New' China Daily." *My Global Eye.* http://myglobaleye. blogspot.co.uk/2009/10/new-china-daily.html.

Henig, R. M. 2002. "The Life and Legacy of Paul de Kruif." *Alicia Patterson Foundation.* http://aliciapatterson.org/stories/life-and-legacy-paul-de-kruif.

Hills, C. 2015. "'I Would like the Last Guinea Worm to Die before I Do.'" *Public Radio International.* https://pri.org/stories/2015-08-21/jimmy-carter-i-would-last-guinea-worm-die-i-do.

Horizon. 2005. "Defeating the Curse Transcript." *BBC Science & Nature*. https://bbc. co.uk/sn/tvradio/programmes/horizon/malaria_trans.shtml.

Hotez, P. 2014a. "Chagas Disease: Urgent Measures Are Needed." *The Huffington Post*. https://huffingtonpost.com/peter-hotez-md-phd/chagas-disease_b_4675010.html.

———. 2014b. "Chagas Disease: A 2014 World Cup Yellow Card." *The Huffington Post*. https://huffingtonpost.com/peter-hotez-md-phd/chagas-disease-2014-world-cup_b_5367793.html.

Hotez, P. J. 2002. "Reducing the Global Burden of Human Parasitic Diseases." *Comparative Parasitology* 69 (2): 140–45. https://doi.org/10.1654/1525-2647 (2002)069[0140:RTGBOH]2.0.CO;2.

———. 2012a. "Tropical Diseases: The New Plague of Poverty." *The New York Times*. https://nytimes.com/2012/08/19/opinion/sunday/tropical-diseases-the-new-plague-of-poverty.html.

Hotez, P. J. 2008. "Reinventing Guantanamo: From Detainee Facility to Center for Research on Neglected Diseases of Poverty in the Americas." *PLoS Neglected Tropical Diseases* 2 (2): e201. https://doi.org/10.1371/journal.pntd.0000201.

———. 2012b. "The Four Horsemen of the Apocalypse: Tropical Medicine in the Fight against Plague, Death, Famine, and War." *The American Journal of Tropical Medicine and Hygiene* 87 (1): 3–10. https://doi.org/10.4269/ajtmh.2012.11-0814.

———. 2013. *Forgotten People Forgotten Diseases*. Edited by Peter J. Hotez. American Society of Microbiology. https://doi.org/10.1128/9781555818753.

———. 2014a. "The Medical Biochemistry of Poverty and Neglect." *Molecular Medicine* 20 (Suppl 1): S31–S6. https://doi.org/10.2119/molmed.2014.00169.

———. 2014b. "Global Christianity and the Control of Its Neglected Tropical Diseases." *PLoS Neglected Tropical Diseases* 8 (11): e3135. https://doi.org/10.1371/journal.pntd.0003135.

———. 2016a. "The South China Sea and Its Neglected Tropical Diseases." *PLoS Neglected Tropical Diseases* 10 (3): e0004395. https://doi.org/10.1371/journal.pntd.0004395.

———. 2016b. "Neglected Tropical Diseases in the Anthropocene: The Cases of Zika, Ebola, and Other Infections." *PLoS Neglected Tropical Diseases* 10 (4): e0004648. https://doi.org/10.1371/journal.pntd.0004648.

Hotez, P. J., & J. P. Ehrenberg. 2010. "Escalating the Global Fight against Neglected Tropical Diseases through Interventions in the Asia Pacific Region." *Advances in Parasitology* 72 (January): 31–53. https://doi.org/10.1016/S0065-308X(10)72002-9.

Hotez, P. J., J. H. F. Remme, P. Buss, G. Alleyne, C. Morel, & J. G. Breman. 2004. "Combating Tropical Infectious Diseases: Report of the Disease Control Priorities in Developing Countries Project." *Clinical Infectious Diseases: An Official Publication of the Infectious Diseases Society of America* 38 (6): 871–78. https://doi.org/10.1086/382077.

Jasanoff, S. 2005. *Designs on Nature: Science and Democracy in Europe and the United States*. Princeton University Press. https://books.google.ca/books/about/Designs_on_Nature.html?id=gUpVtzqtvw0C&pgis=1.

Keating, C. 2014. "Ken Warren and the Rockefeller Foundation's Great Neglected Diseases Network, 1978–1988: The Transformation of Tropical and Global Medicine." *Molecular Medicine* 20 (Suppl 1) (January): S24–S30. https://doi.org/10.2119/molmed.2014.00221.

Klass, P. 2015. "The War on Hookworms." *The New Yorker*. https://newyorker.com/tech/elements/war-of-the-worms.

Kreier, J. P. 2014. *Malaria: Immunology and Immunization*. Elsevier Science. https://books.google.com/books?id=mJniBQAAQBAJ&pgis=1.

Kropf, S. P., & M. Romero Sá. 2009. "The Discovery of Trypanosoma Cruzi and Chagas Disease (1908–1909): Tropical Medicine in Brazil." *História, Ciências, Saúde-Manguinhos* 16 (July): 13–34. https://doi.org/10.1590/S0104-59702009000500002.

Kruif, P. D. 2002. *Microbe Hunters*. Harcourt Brace. https://books.google.com/books?id=pH24vLpivRgC&pgis=1.

Kupferschmidt, K. 2015. "Discovered a Disease? WHO Has New Rules for Avoiding Offensive Names." *Science*. https://sciencemag.org/news/2015/05/discovered-disease-who-has-new-rules-avoiding-offensive-names.

Lancet. 2009. "What Has the Gates Foundation Done for Global Health?" *The Lancet* 373 (9675): 1577. https://doi.org/10.1016/S0140-6736(09)60885-0.

Lemaine, G., R. Macleod, M. Mulkay, P. Weingart, & W. de Gruyter. 1976. *Perspectives on the Emergence of Scientific Disciplines*. Walter de Gruyter. https://books.google.co.uk/books/about/Perspectives_on_the_Emergence_of_Scienti.html?id=PfotstpTldoC&pgis=1.

Lorenzetti, L. 2016. "Blockbuster Drug Launches 2016: The 7 to Watch." *Fortune*. http://fortune.com/2016/03/25/new-blockbuster-drugs-to-watch/.

Lu, F. C. 1969. "Men against Asian Diseases." *Taiwan Today*. http://taiwantoday.tw/ct.asp?xitem=134607&ctnode=1347&mp=9.

Lucivero, F. 2016. *Ethical Assessments of Emerging Technologies*. The International Library of Ethics, Law and Technology. Cham: Springer International Publishing. https://doi.org/10.1007/978-3-319-23282-9.

Marton, F., P. Fensham, & S. Chaiklin. 1994. "A Nobel's Eye View of Scientific Intuition: Discussions with the Nobel Prize-winners in Physics, Chemistry and Medicine (1970-86)." *International Journal of Science Education* 16 (4): 457–73. https://doi.org/10.1080/0950069940160406.

McKenna, P. 2011. "Nobel Prize goes to modest woman who beat malaria for China" https://newscientist.com/article/mg21228382.000-the-modest-woman-who-beat-malaria-for-china/.

Medline (PubMed) trend. n.d. "Medline Trend: Automated Yearly Statistics of PubMed Results for Any Query." Accessed March 23, 2016. http://dan.corlan.net/medline-trend.html.

Meyer, D. S. 1995. "Framing National Security: Elite Public Discourse on Nuclear Weapons during the Cold War." *Political Communication* 12 (2): 173–92. https://doi.org/10.1080/10584609.1995.9963064.

Miller, L. H., & X. Su. 2011. "Artemisinin: Discovery from the Chinese Herbal Garden." *Cell* 146 (6): 855–58. https://doi.org/10.1016/j.cell.2011.08.024.

Molyneux, D. H., P. J. Hotez, & A. Fenwick. 2005. "'Rapid-Impact Interventions': How a Policy of Integrated Control for Africa's Neglected Tropical Diseases Could Benefit the Poor." *PLoS Medicine* 2 (11): e336. https://doi.org/10.1371/journal.pmed.0020336.

Molyneux, DD. H., & S. A. Ward. 2015. "Reflections on the Nobel Prize for Medicine 2015—The Public Health Legacy and Impact of Avermectin and Artemisinin." *Trends in Parasitology* 31 (12): 605–7. https://doi.org/10.1016/j.pt.2015.10.008.

Morel, C. M. 1999. "Chagas Disease, from Discovery to Control - and beyond: History, Myths and Lessons to Take Home." *Memórias Do Instituto Oswaldo Cruz* 94 (Suppl 1) (January): 3–16. https://ncbi.nlm.nih.gov/pubmed/10677688.

NDTV. 2013. "When Diseases Have a Bad Name, Change Is Hard." New Delhi Television (NDTV). https://ndtv.com/world-news/when-diseases-have-a-bad-name-change-is-hard-536374.

Nightingale, P., & P. Martin. 2004. "The Myth of the Biotech Revolution." *Trends in Biotechnology* 22 (11): 564–69. https://doi.org/10.1016/j.tibtech.2004.09.010.

Nobel Prize. n.d. "Alfred Nobel's Will." https://nobelprize.org/alfred_nobel/will/.

Nordrum, A. 2015. "How Three Scientists 'Marketed' Neglected Tropical Diseases and Raised More Than \$1 Billion | Global Network."| *IBT Times*. https://ibtimes.com/how-three-scientists-marketed-neglected-tropical-diseases-raised-more-1-billion-1921008.

Parker, M., & T. Allen. 2011. "Does Mass Drug Administration for the Integrated Treatment of Neglected Tropical Diseases Really Work? Assessing Evidence for the Control of Schistosomiasis and Soil-Transmitted Helminths in Uganda." *Health Research Policy and Systems/BioMed Central* 9 (1): 3. https://doi.org/10.1186/1478-4505-9-3.

Pathak, D. 2014. "Dr. Peter Hotez Named U.S. Science Envoy." *Baylor College of Medicine News*. https://bcm.edu/news/awards-honors-faculty-staff/dr-peter-hotez-named-us-science-envoy.

Pincock, S. 2011. "Paulo Buss - a Leader of Public Health and Health Policy in Brazil." *The Lancet* 377 (9779): 1738. https://doi.org/10.1016/S0140-6736(11)60719-8.

Polanyi, M. 1962. "The Republic of Science: Its Political and Economic Theory." *Minerva* 38 (1): 1–21. https://doi.org/10.1023/A:1026591624255.

Regnier, M. 2012a. "Neglected Tropical Diseases: A New Handle on Old Problems | Wellcome Trust Blog on WordPress.Com."| *Wellcome Trust*. http://blog.wellcome.ac.uk/2012/01/06/neglected-tropical-diseases-new-handle-old-problems/.

———. 2012b. "Neglected Tropical Diseases: The Campaign Trail." *Wellcome Trust*. http://blog.wellcome.ac.uk/2012/01/10/neglected-tropical-diseases-the-campaign-trail/.

Relman, D., & E. Choffnes. 2010. "Infectious Disease Movement in a Borderless World: Workshop Summary." *Books.Google.Com* 1–323.

Remme, J. H. F., E. Blas, L. Chitsulo, P. M. P. Desjeux, H. D. Engers, T. P. Kanyok, J. F. Kengeya Kayondo, et al. 2002. "Strategic Emphases for Tropical Diseases Research: A TDR Perspective." *Trends in Parasitology* 18 (10): 421–26. https://doi.org/10.1016/S1471-4922(02)02387-5.

Saporta, M. 2012. "An Amazing Tale of Three Men and a Miracle Drug Changing Lives of Millions." *Saporta Report*. http://saportareport.com/an-amazing-tale-of-how-three-men-and-a-miracle-drug-changed-millions-of-lives/.

Savioli, L., A. Montresor, & A. F. Gabrielli. 2011. *Neglected Tropical Diseases: The Development of a Brand with No Copyright: A Shift from a Disease-Centred to a Tool Centred Strategic Approach*. National Academies Press. https://ncbi.nlm.nih.gov/books/NBK62524/.

Scheinberg, I. H. & J. M. Walshe. 1989. *Orphan Diseases and Orphan Drugs*. Manchester University Press. https://books.google.com/books?id=ORkNAQAAIAAJ&pgis=1.

Shakur, R. 2005. "A Professor of Tropical Medicine and Infectious Diseases." *BMJ Careers*. http://careers.bmj.com/careers/advice/view-article.html?id=719.

Singh, A. R., & S. A. Singh. 2008. "Diseases of Poverty and Lifestyle, Well-Being and Human Development." *Mens Sana Monographs* 6 (1): 187–225. https://doi.org/10.4103/0973-1229.40567.

Smith, R. 2014. "Richard Smith: Rebranding and Telling Stories about NCD." *BMJ Blogs*. http://blogs.bmj.com/bmj/2014/06/03/richard-smith-rebranding-and-telling-stories-about-ncd/.

Sternberg, S. 2009. "This Scientist's Passion: Ending the Scourge of Parasitic Diseases." *USA Today*. http://usatoday30.usatoday.com/news/health/2009-03-23-hotez-parasitic-diseases_N.htm.

Stoll, N. R. 1947. "This Wormy World." *The Journal of Parasitology* 33 (1): 1–18. https://ncbi.nlm.nih.gov/pubmed/20284977.

Taylor, H. R. 2008. *Trachoma: A Blinding Scourge from the Bronze Age to the Twenty-First Century*. Haddington Press Australia. http://iehu.unimelb.edu.au/__data/assets/pdf_file/0009/719649/Trachoma_Book_HRTaylor.pdf.

The Rockefeller Foundation. 1978. "The Rockefeller Foundation Annual Report." RF Annual Report. 1978. https://rockefellerfoundation.org/app/uploads/Annual-Report-1978.pdf.

The Rockefeller University. n.d. "History of The Rockefeller University." https://rockefeller.edu/about/history.

Wang, Z. 2002. "Saving China through Science: The Science Society of China, Scientific Nationalism, and Civil Society in Republican China." *Osiris* 17 (1): 291–322. https://doi.org/10.1086/649367.

Warren, K. S., & Bowers J. D. 1982. *Parasitology: A Global Perspective*. Springer Science & Business Media. https://books.google.com/books?id=CVjSBwAAQBAJ&pgis=1.

Warren, K. S. 1978. "Hepatosplenic Schistosomiasis: A Great Neglected Disease of the Liver." *Gut* 19 (6): 572–77. https://doi.org/10.1136/gut.19.6.572.

WHO. 2007. "Global Plan to Combat Neglected Tropical Diseases 2008–2015." http://apps.who.int/iris/bitstream/10665/69708/1/WHO_CDS_NTD_2007.3_eng.pdf.

———. 2010. "First WHO Report on Neglected Tropical Diseases: Working to Overcome the Global Impact of Neglected Tropical Diseases." https://who.int/neglected_diseases/2010report/en/.

———. 2012. "Accelerating Work to Overcome the Global Impact of Neglected Tropical Diseases: A Roadmap for Implementation: Executive Summary." http://apps.who.int//iris/handle/10665/70809.

———. 2015. "World Health Organization Best Practices for the Naming of New Human Infectious Diseases." https://who.int/publications/i/item/WHO-HSE-FOS-15.1.

———. 2016. "Report of the WHO Strategic and Technical Advisory Group for Neglected Tropical Diseases." https://who.int/neglected_diseases/NTD_STAG_report_2015.pdf.

Yang, G., L. Liu, H. Zhu, S. M Griffiths, M. Tanner, R. Bergquist, J. Utzinger, & X. Zhou. 2014. "China's Sustained Drive to Eliminate Neglected Tropical Diseases." *The Lancet. Infectious Diseases* 14 (9): 881–92. https://doi.org/10.1016/S1473-3099(14)70727-3.

Zhou, X. 2013. "China's Experience Controlling Neglected Tropical Disease and the Lessons for Other Regions." *Duke Global Health Institute.* http://globalhealth.duke.edu/media/blogs/china/chinas-experience-controlling- neglected-tropical-disease-and-lessons-other-regions.

Chapter 6

Conclusion
Neglect in policy

Policy rationales

Understanding the meaning behind the use of measurement and advocacy in policy has required specific attention to the assumptions, practices, and implications of neglect for NTDs policy. The introduction set the background for how NTDs have become a label for a group of diseases, previously called tropical diseases, positioned next to the 'Big Three' – HIV/AIDS, TB, and malaria – that have dominated in global health. Chapter 2 presented the theory on approaching policy problems, to make sense of the 'who, what, why, and where' that leads to a topic being considered as a problem for policy. Conceptions of neglect build on recent sociological research into ignorance and absences, differently characterised through the addition of implicit blame and responsibility, between neglector and neglected. Chapter 3 provided a view of the key events in a timeline for the policy development of NTDs that led to commitments from the Gates Foundation and big pharma donations, as well as the early conceptualisation of NTDs through the Special Programme for Research and Training in Tropical Diseases (TDR) and the Great Neglected Diseases of Mankind (GND).

Chapter 4 returned to categorisation to take a longer historical look into how NTDs transitioned from tropical diseases, through the colonial history legacy and current geography, in determining 'what is tropical?' and 'what is neglected?'. The answer is shown to be largely described through ideas of poverty and underdevelopment, leading to a dominant drug-based strategy for intervention. Chapter 5 showed how neglect is imagined through a globalised policy for NTDs that arises from a position of 'otherness' and is based on an ultimate goal of eradication, but does not consider endemic country needs well when neglect is understood in mainly universal terms. NTDs form a disease brand to recharacterise tropical diseases, and I profiled scientist advocates in the US, UK, Brazil, and China.

This final chapter again returns to question how 'otherness' plays a persistent role in the tropical medicine project from an early stage. Edmond describes how "(A)s Europe slowly freed itself from an epidemiological past of cholera, malaria, leprosy and plague, these and other diseases were banished to the tropics where they became a primary signifier of native otherness" (Edmond, 2006, pp. 117–8). Iris Marion Young (2011) also warns against a binary distinction between dominating and dominated groups, but views domination as a structural phenomenon. Otherness results from fluid and complex relations that may be unconscious and even arbitrary, but is a situation of privilege produced from unequal structures. In other social spheres that neglect is seen in, who is doing the dominating may be more or less obvious, one responsible party over another. Examples are neglect of children by their parents or guardians, elder neglect of the elderly by their carers or family, animal neglect of pets, farming or working animals by their owners, and environmental neglect of buildings or nature.

To understand how domination and otherness both causes and results in neglect, it is worth recalling the object of enquiry this book set out upon. The WHO outlines 20 'neglected' tropical diseases as being in need of attention and deeply affecting health in poor communities. Progress is being made: two diseases are targets for eradication (guinea worm and yaws), and eight more are marked for regional and global elimination (trachoma, Chagas disease, African sleeping sickness, leishmaniases, lymphatic filariasis, river blindness, rabies, and schistosomiasis), and in 2018, eight countries eliminated at least one NTD (WHO, 2019). As noted previously, elimination relates to a defined geographic area where disease transmission is interrupted, while eradication requires global co-operation to rid humankind of a disease completely (Hopkins, 2011, p. 19). Elimination and eradication become closely and conceptually tied with neglect, and the very idea is ideological. The solution for neglect of diseases, from this perspective, is to eradicate the disease as a medical problem and not to focus on social, political, and economic circumstances that may be underlying causes.

Stepan argues that eradication has been historically a part of an imperial view of tropical medicine (2013, p. 7). Now it carries weight with the technology solutionism of big pharma and the technocratic Bill and Melinda Gates Foundation. While NTDs are at various stages on the path to eradication, the end point appears close but not yet met. If this pursuit is ideological, from a position of domination, the importance also of control, surveillance, or even short-term measures must also be considered as they tend to be deprioritised in favour of a long-term goal of eradication. Reviewing the dominant strategies to deal with NTDs suggests that it is not the case that long-term goals are prioritised as the availability of cheap drugs to control NTDs on a short-term basis is central. However, there are other non-medical factors that also contribute to the persistence of NTDs.

Social, political, and economic factors that create and perpetuate disease that are sometimes summarised as the 'social determinants of health', have reached mainstream public health policy to address inequities, evidenced by

WHO reporting, task groups, and commitments (WHO, 2014). However, neglect in a policy sense should be understood differently in the differing attention and competition between global health problems.

A typology of neglect

As noted in the introduction, this book has been concerned with advocacy and measurement in the development of policy problems across political sites of global health. Advocacy and measurement from the side of the neglectors, has had a tremendous impact upon diseases of the poorest and most vulnerable. Thus, the actors and circumstances directing policy was the focus of this book. Advocacy has been central through a concerted backing of NTDs through scientist advocates. Measurement, in addition to advocacy, was needed to make a case for caring, through measurement metrics to assess the scale of a problem and provide proof for economic development outcomes for health.

What then has this study of advocacy and measurement contributed to an understanding of neglect in policy? NTDs are defined firstly by what they are not, as the opposite of attention and care. A multitude of descriptors point towards the reasons; and through this research, a typology of neglect has emerged. In suggesting a typology it was important not to fall into the trap of what McGoey describes in ignorance studies as trying to address "immeasurable ways of saying nothing" (2012, p. 7). Applying scales of neglect would be a difficult undertaking to qualify, but types of neglect is something I observed for the problem understanding and solutions proposed forming opposites to acknowledgement, to attention, and to care. Neglect as a policy characterisation in the NTD case has spanned emotional neglect, informational neglect, neglect of thought, and neglect to act as contributions to the understanding of policy problems.

This typology has some similarities with four components that Nimmo outlined in his 1974 book '*Popular Images of Politics: A Taxonomy*', in how an image of a policy problem is projected and perceived. He identifies how an image is represented as being perceptual (through direct observation or a processing of information), affective (with feeling or emotion), cognitive (in interpretation or thought), and conative (for action potential) (ibid., p. 9). Nimmo's typology has had limited influence outside of political campaigning and communication scholarship, but there are parallels with how political images are represented and perceived, and how policy problems are understood and responded to. Figure 6.1 shows neglect as being grouped across four aspects: neglect in information, emotion, thought, and action. 'Emotional neglect' and 'neglect in action' are shown as more connected with an advocacy response; and 'informational neglect' and 'neglect of thought' are shown as closely related to a measurement response to produce evidence.

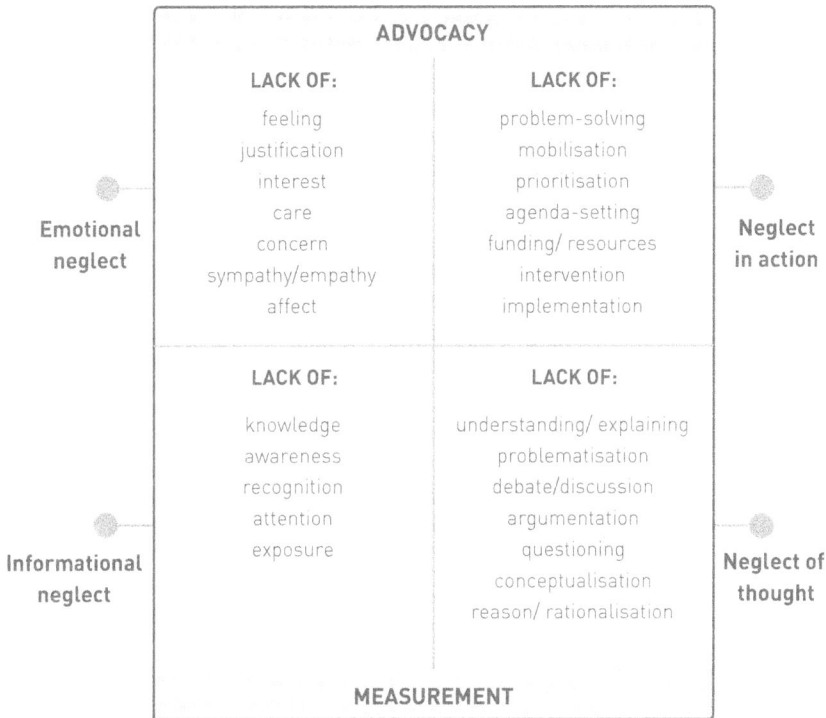

Figure 6.1 A typology of neglect in policy.

Information

Information and informational arguments are used to persuade or rank and can be considered as being a first step to provoking emotion, action, and thought (although activity might also be spurred through the action of social movements or thought applied to an issue). If information is lacking, or what is used to inform policy is not supportive, a policy problem may have difficulty in getting traction. Information is used through the metrics to measure neglect and present evidence on NTDs. Informational neglect may be uneven, depending upon who is finding and presenting the information. It is taken as given that not everyone possesses equal information and it is a further question as to whether it is the right information (Wankhade & Dabade, 2010).

Emotion

Kenneth Warren, the director of the GND, described epidemiology as "… compassion with the tears wiped away" (Keating, 2014, p. S29), which implies how emotion has been viewed as to somehow degrade serious thought and work. However, as a topic of study, emotion has seen an entry as a driving force in response to social issues. Sympathy or empathy is an emotional connection to an issue, which causes attention, interest, awareness, and recognition, or, more strongly, concern and care. Emotion has been devalued as a persuasion tool and seen to interfere with the measurement of impact and effectiveness, but despite a contentious status, emotion remains closely tied to philanthropy and public health. Emotional neglect played a part in response to the HIV/AIDS crisis through the 'emotions work' that was needed to persuade people to care (Gould, 2009). Care, as an emotion of concern or interest, is also a defining feature of public health. This spans from micro-level caring for the sick to the macro of caring for populations and caring about what makes them sick.

Action

Lack of action may appear to be a straightforward form of neglect. Social movements exemplify action, but there are also alternative forms, through policy advocacy. Other ways of describing policy action in the literature have been through 'modes of co-ordination' or 'regimes of action' (Jessop, 1999). The ways in which caring in global health is connected to action through the ability or capacity to care is described by David Reubi et al.:

> The ability and will to care, in turn, is shaped by the complex, multi-scalar politics and resource flows that condition so much of the global health enterprise. Care implies a need for empathy, responsibility and duty just as much as it does the fair distribution of medical services and resources and the capacity to access and make use of these.
>
> (Reubi et al., 2015, p. 4)

Care is not possible without being able to act – to be able to distribute medical services and resources, and provide fair access. Much of the effort to create the NTD brand took place in the UK and US, as places of 'high politics' of global health (Storeng & Béhague, 2014, p. 266). It should be noted that a spotlight on this activity through media attention, and the skew towards the UK and US in main events and milestones,[1] have meant that the actions of endemic countries have not been well acknowledged.

Thought

Responding to a global health problem is not only grounded in action, information, and emotion, but in thought, too. This is the thoughtful reflection of what problems mean, what is involved, and what is at stake. The literature on policy problems indicates that 'thought' is analytically putting information to work, whether it is to present arguments, structure discussions and debates, or to problematise issues. For NTDs, thought has been the conceptual work on the brand and the accompanying policy rationale. It is presumed to put to use reason, rationality, and morality, but can also be an argumentative activity involving justification and rationale that is both emotional and thought-based.

Some of the responses to neglect clearly cut across type, and there may be overlap. There is a danger in perpetuating dualities or dichotomies (e.g. between emotion and information already discussed) and potentially drawing lines where they do not truly exist. Therefore, this typology is a heuristic to question what is meant by neglect and an acknowledgement that, in sorting meaning, we actively place ideas into camps. More widely, this typology seeks an expansion of enquiry for the sociological study of absence and ignorance of problems which pertain in the main to a lack of or suppression of information (and associated knowledge).

Who is responsible?

Responsibility lies behind information, action, emotion, and thought for NTDs. But where does it lie and with whom? For issues where neglect has become a synonymous characterisation, responsibility may appear clearer. For example, medical neglect takes place on an individual basis with a doctor's or hospital's failure of a duty of care to a patient. Sometimes responsibility can also fall on individuals for not caring for their health adequately (e.g. illness related to obesity or smoking) (Herrick, 2009) or wider institutional, governmental, and societal reasons that make medical neglect systematic. Responsibility can shift, as with drug and alcohol abuse; blame can be a moral judgment of behaviour or blamed on being an illness (Martin, 1999).

The agency assigned to the neglected party becomes central. Child and elder neglect are more obvious examples, as the neglected are viewed as weaker and more vulnerable, with a duty of care from the parents, guardians, or carers. However, child abuse and neglect had to be accepted as a concept (Hacking, 1991) before legal protection and recompense was possible. The first legal case of physical child abuse occurred in 1874, but as the concept had not yet found a legal form, it had to be brought forward by the American Society for the Prevention of Cruelty to Animals (Markel, 2009).[2] It is an example of how neglect can also be systemic in legal, policy, political, cultural, or social systems. Similarly, the label of neglect was required for the policy problem of NTDs to be identified and dealt with.

NTDs are a complicated proposition on which to assign blame because of the many societal actors involved. More generally, societal neglect is a failure to care when one should, and it may include all societal actors, with varying responsibilities. Responsibility for health can be thought of as being grouped into the following major areas: personal, governmental, social, and environmental (Collins, 2004). The social and environmental perspective has gained ground through the rise of epidemiology, looking at health of populations and the governmentality of the populace with responsibility for health placed with the state. Balance between personal and societal responsibility moves back and forth, as well as how epidemiology is interested in individual risk factors of disease and government taxes 'unhealthy' individuals (e.g. through sugar, alcohol, and cigarettes).

If responsibility is spread amongst various actors, as with NTDs, this returns to the question of how it is divided, whether equally or to varying degrees. Big pharma is thought to supply the drugs and innovation or R&D. Whether or not they need incentives to do so is debated, as has who pays – the donation of drugs was not straightforwardly arrived at. Similarly, governments of donor countries and international organisations such as the UN have provided most of the funding for NTDs. Funding has more lately switched to philanthropic foundations, including the Gates Foundation and endemic countries themselves, especially middle-income countries such as Brazil and China.

The expectations of various actors will also change, as big pharma is expected to have a larger corporate social responsibility role, and governments are expected to provide more than access and encompass: "… sanitation, pollution control, food and drug safety, health education, disease surveillance, urban planning and occupational health" (Resnik, 2007, p. 444). Although I have presented how neglect can be thought of as lacking across four areas (information, emotion, action, and thought), simply identifying types of neglect does not assign agency or causality, nor answer why neglect occurs.

NTDs today: taking out the 'neglect'

What, then, are the perceived conceptual weaknesses and future research directions for neglect, in order to go beyond the case of NTDs? A first consideration to make is that NTDs do not have the monopoly on neglect in global health, despite their name. Neglect can also be part of being a high-profile disease. The relationship between NTDs and the Big Three has been a constant theme. Malaria, the non-neglected tropical disease, is exemplary of the continuum of neglect that diseases exist on, until the event of control, elimination, or (unlikely) eradication. As Kelly and Beisel describe:

> Despite that attention, neglect remains central to malaria's high profile. After the first malaria eradication campaign was abandoned in the late 1960s, funding for malaria-specific health interventions decreased dramatically, causing case numbers to soar … That narrative of abandonment and resurgence, we suggest, is linked to a military industrial concern: an all-or-nothing commitment that links health advances to

technological innovation and pathogen-obliteration, constituting malaria anew along untapped markets and neglected fronts.

(2011, p. 72)

What did it mean for malaria to be neglected, un-neglected, and then neglected again, with the characterisation as such? Viewing malaria alongside NTDs, neglect is a part of the attention that diseases received in the past, how attention has accelerated, and then regressed again. The way of dealing with neglect in the case of malaria appears to be all-out warfare, where either everything is thrown in or nothing.[3] As such, neglect is an enigmatic and increasingly used concept in policy to identify global problems. A second consideration is what is left when an issue once labelled as neglected is no longer neglected? As Sudeepa Abeysinghe (2015) argues, ignorance claims about NTDs are a call to action. It is not only claims on the grounds of information that invoke action, as I have shown through the typology of neglect; ignorance (through lack of knowledge or information) is only one-part corrected by addressing neglect. Claims are made on aspects of neglect on the grounds of emotion, thought, and action, but all may not be addressed equally.

What, then, will happen if all aspects of neglect are addressed? The characterisation of neglect is an ongoing process, but what is next when it reaches a desired end-point? This is part paradox of language, as to call something neglected can be reasonable from the outset but then become contradictory as it reaches a conclusion, with the term being used more and the issue addressed. The strategic power of the 'neglect' label as a discursive construct can be diminished or even become detrimental; and if this happened, the question would remain as to what would replace it? The need for a straightforward and cohesive policy transformation of disease is inherently problematic. NTDs could no longer be neglected, but that does not mean the problem is solved, as action taken may be ineffective, counterproductive, or even cause unintended adverse consequences. Therefore, the characterisation of neglect will not necessarily mean that NTDs are dealt with in the best way possible.

Furthermore, truly neglected issues and topics may be those that are not identified as such in the first place, as found in the sociological absence and ignorance literature; or some policy problems are not addressed because they are judged not to be neglected enough but require ongoing or new types of support. This quandary of neglect can be demonstrated further through emerging diseases (HIV/AIDS, Ebola, and COVID-19), re-emerging diseases (as a threat, it was not previously seen with dengue and Zika), and persistent diseases (malaria and polio, with polio continuing to be elusively close to eradication). Neglect rarely reaches an end point in global health – only smallpox comes close, eradicated from the world. Even then, there is a continued threat, and it can also have uses – for example, in research.

Emergence and re-emergence are related topics to neglected and un-neglected in policy problems, pertinent to global health. Emergence relates to the increase in incidence of a disease, but also whether it is recognised, while neglect more specifically relates to the policy reaction and implies that it is not enough or insufficient in some way. The compulsion to create categories to place diseases into does not appear to be diminishing. According to the WHO, an emerging disease is "... one that has appeared in a population for the first time, or that may have existed previously but is rapidly increasing in incidence or geographic range" (WHO, n.d.). The fear of emerging diseases and interest in this category does not look to decrease soon, and this clearly has an intimate relationship with neglect, existing in a world of already established health priorities, disease hierarchies, and competing policy agendas.

A number of outbreaks and epidemics have arisen from diseases originating in poor communities in tropical and semi-tropical regions, but with global implications. However, interest in these diseases is also connected to how they affect more affluent countries. Indeed, the Ebola outbreak opened a door for dialogue on wider lessons for global health security (Heymann et al., 2015).[4] Jackson and Stephenson (2014) similarly view a connection between NTDs and emerging infectious diseases as being socio-political constructs. They view the neglect of NTDs on humanitarian terms, an argument that is seldom made for these diseases, apart from at the beginning of their construction in the early WHO reports, stating: "We suggest that 'neglect' reflects the rise of a secular humanitarian global health moral not only in the Global North but more pervasively" (ibid., p. 997). Therefore, neglect materialises when considering health as a global moral duty deserving of humanitarian intervention. Instead of repeating the 'right to health' humanitarian approach, Jackson and Stephenson (2014) invoke action to address neglect as part of the 'right to development'. This approach is a symbiosis of the dominant economic development approach and the mostly disregarded humanitarian approach to NTDs on the global stage. Rather than a view of health in times of emergency, the everyday reality of health is employed for the priorities of international security, design of global infrastructures, and the practices of global governance.

Political theorists such as Joao Nunes (2013) have been considering how health problems can be constructed in certain ways,[5] as he argues for Zika: "While the world is only now beginning to see Zika as an emergency, the conditions that have enabled the spread of the virus and hindered response are 'everyday emergencies' for millions of Brazilians" (2013). Nunes, with other researchers, is interested in the impact of technical instruments and scientific practices that permeate international affairs (Mayer et al., 2014). More recently, Simukai Chigudu has commented on the inevitability of communicable disease in Africa in the context of COVID-19:

> Contrasting the horror of COVID-19 in the Global North with its
> presumed trajectory in Africa offers an important yet ignored political

question about how and why the suffering induced by communicable diseases is treated as unthinkable in one place and inevitable in another.

(Langstaff, 2020)

This book has made a step towards analysing neglect as an important concept for understanding policy problems, both in terms of how actors use neglect to make problem claims and also for unravelling the dynamics that allow policy issues to rise in prominence or not. Neglect in policy is not to know (information), not to care (emotion), not to think about (thought), and not to act on (action). All social actors in global health are implicated and responsible to varying degrees, but it is under these constraints that advocacy through scientist advocates, and evidence in the production and use of measurement metrics, have come about. As an in-depth study of NTDs, this research can be absorbed within sociology of absences and ignorance literature to make for a more encompassing view of neglect in policy, while forming part of a future agenda in the critical consideration of how policy problems compete, rise in prominence, and coincide.

Notes

1   The first NTD paper, Global Network, London Declaration, Presidential Initiative on NTDs and DFID commitment.
2   Now child neglect cases are reported as the most frequent form of child abuse (NSPCC, https://nspcc.org.uk/preventing-abuse/child-abuse-and-neglect/neglect/, accessed 2/4/2014).
3   Closely related is memory and amnesia. These are forgotten events, places, people, a collective amnesia, purposeful, or accidental, "… cycles of public health amnesia, memory and neglect" (ibid., p. 71).
4   As David Heymann has highlighted, attention to collective health security is not enough. We also need to acknowledge individual health security: "This is security that comes from access to safe and effective health services, products, and technologies" (ibid., p. 1884). The idea of collective health security has dominated in international relations, with the focus being on contagion of infectious diseases across countries, where the political impact of disease across countries is one of emergency. Note: some tropical diseases do involve vectors that travel (e.g. dengue) and people who move with disease (e.g. Chagas) (Hotez, 2014).
5   This is a consideration of the intentions of international actors, their relations with one another, as well as overarching international policy trends. The characterisation of disease and rationales for intervention become spheres of contestation and collaboration between countries, and for the negotiation of policy.

References

Abeysinghe, S. 2015. "Ignorance Claims as a Call to Action: The Case of Neglected Tropical Diseases." Working Paper. https://icpublicpolicy.org/conference/file/reponse/1433940937.pdf.

Collins, K. 2004. "Profitable Gifts: A History of the Merck Mectizan Donation Program and Its Implications for International Health." *Perspectives in Biology and Medicine* 47 (1): 100–9. https://ncbi.nlm.nih.gov/pubmed/15061171.

Edmond, R. 2006. *Leprosy and Empire*. Cambridge: Cambridge University Press. https://doi.org/10.1017/CBO9780511497285.

Gould, D. B. 2009. *Moving Politics: Emotion and Act up's Fight against AIDS*. University of Chicago Press.

Hacking, I. 1991. "The Making and Molding of Child Abuse." *Critical Inquiry* 17 (2): 253–88. https://doi.org/10.1086/448583.

Herrick, C. 2009. "Shifting Blame/Selling Health: Corporate Social Responsibility in the Age of Obesity." *Sociology of Health & Illness* 31 (1): 51–65. https://doi.org/10.1111/j.1467-9566.2008.01121.x.

Heymann, D. L., L. Chen, K. Takemi, D. P. Fidler, J. W. Tappero, M. J. Thomas, T. A. Kenyon, et al. 2015. "Global Health Security: The Wider Lessons from the West African Ebola Virus Disease Epidemic." *The Lancet* 385 (9980): 1884–1901. https://doi.org/10.1016/S0140-6736(15)60858-3.

Hopkins, D. R. 2011. Neglected Tropical Diseases (NTDs) Slated for Elimination and Eradication. *National Academies Press (US)*. Retrieved from https://ncbi.nlm.nih.gov/books/NBK62516/.

Hotez, P. 2014, January 28. Chagas Disease: Urgent Measures Are Needed. *The Huffington Post*. Retrieved from https://huffingtonpost.com/peter-hotez-md-phd/chagas-disease_b_4675010.html.

Jackson, Y., & N. Stephenson. 2014. "Neglected Tropical Disease and Emerging Infectious Disease: An Analysis of the History, Promise and Constraints of Two Worldviews." *Global Public Health* 9 (9): 995–1007. https://doi.org/10.1080/17441692.2014.941297.

Jessop, B. 1999. "The Changing Governance of Welfare: Recent Trends in Its Primary Functions, Scale, and Modes of Coordination." *Social Policy and Administration* 33 (4): 348–59. https://doi.org/10.1111/1467-9515.00157.

Keating, C. 2014. "Ken Warren and the Rockefeller Foundation's Great Neglected Diseases Network, 1978–1988: The Transformation of Tropical and Global Medicine." *Molecular Medicine* 20 (Suppl 1) (January): S24–S30. https://doi.org/10.2119/molmed.2014.00221.

Kelly, A. H., & U. Beisel. 2011. "Neglected Malarias: The Frontlines and Back Alleys of Global Health." *BioSocieties* 6 (S1): 71–87. https://doi.org/10.1057/biosoc.2010.42.

Langstaff, A. 2020. "Pandemic Narratives and the Historian." *The Los Angeles Review of Books*. https://lareviewofbooks.org/article/pandemic-narratives-and-the-historian/.

Markel, H. 2009. "1874 Case of Mary Ellen McCormack Shined First Light on Child Abuse." *The New York Times*. https://nytimes.com/2009/12/15/health/15abus.html.

Martin, M. W. 1999. "Alcoholism as Sickness and Wrongdoing." *Journal for the Theory of Social Behaviour* 29 (2): 109–31. https://doi.org/10.1111/1468-5914.00094.

Mayer, M., M. Carpes, & R. Knoblich. 2014. *The Global Politics of Science and Technology – Vol. 1: Concepts from International Relations and Other Disciplines*. Springer. https://books.google.com/books?id=V7RTBAAAQBAJ&pgis=1.

McGoey, L. 2012. "Strategic Unknowns: Towards a Sociology of Ignorance." *Economy and Society* 41 (1): 1–16. https://doi.org/10.1080/03085147.2011.637330.

Nimmo, D. D. 1974. *Popular Images of Politics: A Taxonomy*. Prentice-Hall.

NSPCC. n.d. "Child Neglect." https://nspcc.org.uk/preventing-abuse/child-abuse-and-neglect/neglect/.

Nunes, J. 2013. *Security, Emancipation and the Politics of Health: A New Theoretical Perspective*. Routledge. https://books.google.com/books?id=YfohAQAAQBAJ&pgis=1.

Resnik, D. B. 2007. "Responsibility for Health: Personal, Social, and Environmental." *Journal of Medical Ethics* 33 (8): 444–45. https://doi.org/10.1136/jme.2006.017574.

Reubi, D., C. Herrick, & T. Brown. 2015. "The Politics of Non-Communicable Diseases in the Global South." *Health & Place* 39: 179–87. https://doi.org/10.1016/j.healthplace.2015.09.001.

Stepan, N. L. 2013. *Eradication: Ridding the World of Diseases Forever?* Reaktion Books. Retrieved from https://books.google.com/books?hl=en&lr=&id=hrleAgAAQBAJ&pgis=1.

Storeng, K. T., & D. P. Béhague. 2014. "Playing the Numbers Game: Evidence-Based Advocacy and the Technocratic Narrowing of the Safe Motherhood Initiative." *Medical Anthropology Quarterly* 28 (2): 260–79. https://doi.org/10.1111/maq.12072.

Wankhade, L., & B. Dabade. 2010. *Quality Uncertainty and Perception: Information Asymmetry and Management of Quality Uncertainty and Quality Perception*. Physica-Verlag.

WHO. n.d. "Emerging Diseases." Accessed February 1, 2016. https://who.int/topics/emerging_diseases/en/.

———. 2014. "Review of Social Determinants and the Health Divide in the WHO European Region. Final Report."

———. 2019. "Defeating Neglected Tropical Diseases. Progress, Challenges and Opportunities." https://who.int/neglected_diseases/resources/who-cds-ntd-2019.01/en/.

Young, I. M. 2011. *Justice and the Politics of Difference*. Princeton University Press.

Index

For Product Safety Concerns and Information please contact our EU
representative GPSR@taylorandfrancis.com
Taylor & Francis Verlag GmbH, Kaufingerstraße 24, 80331 München, Germany

9 7 8 1 0 3 2 0 6 0 7 6 7